NICHOLAS CULPEPER

Nicholas Culpeper

English Physician and Astrologer

OLAV THULESIUS

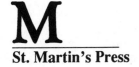

St. Martin's Press

First published in Great Britain 1992 by
THE MACMILLAN PRESS LTD
Houndmills, Basingstoke, Hampshire RG21 2XS
and London
Companies and representatives
throughout the world

A catalogue record for this book is available
from the British Library

ISBN 0–333–55564–3

Printed in Hong Kong

First published in the United States of America 1992 by
Scholarly and Reference Division,
ST. MARTIN'S PRESS, INC.,
175 Fifth Avenue,
New York, N.Y. 10010

ISBN 0–312–07543–X

Library of Congress Cataloging-in-Publication Data
Thulesius, Olav.
Nicholas Culpeper, English physician and astrologer / Olav
Thulesius.
    p. cm.
Includes bibliographical references and index.
ISBN 0–312–07543–X
1. Culpeper, Nicholas, 1616–1654.   2. Herbalists—Great Britain—
Biography.   3. Astrologers—Great Britain—Biography.   I. Title.
RS164.T55   1992
610'.92—dc20
[B]   91–32276
                                                          CIP

Affectionately dedicated to my wife
Layla
whose faithful devotion has helped
to bring this book to a conclusion

Contents

List of Plates

List of Figures

Preface

Two factors prompted my interest in Nicholas Culpeper: my heritage and my profession. I come from a family of apothecaries and from the country and county of Carl von Linné, the great Swedish botanist. I was brought up with the tradition of apothecary jars and pressed flowers. As a physician and teacher of medical students I found it helpful by way of introduction to say a few words about the origin of drugs from herbs. With this background I browsed in the antiquarian bookshops of London and found my first Culpepers: nicely illustrated 19th-century herbals and various facsimile editions. Who was this 17th-century man whose herbal was reprinted as late as 1983? I immediately made the reflection that he certainly must have been an important English physician. However, to my surprise I found no biography of him. At the British Library I found an astonishingly large number of titles *by* Nicholas Culpeper but still very few facts about his short and stormy life. From that time on I began to piece together a picture of the man and his life whenever I was in England, which fortunately happened to be quite often.

The staff of the British Library, the Wellcome Historical Medical Library and the Library of the Royal Society of London have been extremely helpful. Special thanks go to Dr J. De Lima, Mr J. Ayres, Mr M. Phelbs for books and references; and to Rev R. C. Dalling, Major O'Leary and Mrs J. Buckeridge of Isfield, for introducing me to the background of Nicholas Culpeper's childhood in Sussex.

I am also grateful to Steven Gerrard and Anthony Grahame for their assistance in publishing this book.

OLAV THULESIUS
Kuwait and Linköping, 1991

1
Birth in Ockley

Children sweeten labours but they make misfortunes more bitter.

Francis Bacon, 1561–1626

Sixteen hundred and sixteen, in the reign of King James I, was a fateful year – the year in which William Shakespeare died and William Harvey described the circulation of the blood for the first time in his lectures.[1]

On October 18th, a baby boy, Nicholas, was born to Mary and Nicholas Culpeper, the rector of Ockley in Surrey.[2] His father never came to see his son, because he suddenly died before the birth of his only child and was buried on October 5th, 1616 in St Margaret's churchyard. Little Nicholas junior, son of the late parson, was baptised in the same church on October 24th. His grief-stricken mother decided to give him the same name as his father and great-great grandfather, Nicholas. Although this certainly was because of family tradition and sentimental feelings, it became a name very appropriate to his character, Nicholas being the patron saint of the young and the scholars.

This tragic event left a young bereaved widow all alone. Today St Margaret's remains as it was three centuries ago. In the churchyard stand many head stones and old tombs, like little houses. Inscriptions, hardly visible, have been washed away and overgrown by moss, and only rose-trees from centuries past bear witness to the departed loved ones. They were planted here in memory of sweethearts and relatives, a pretty tradition of bygone Surrey.[3]

After the premature death of Nicholas Culpeper, Mary had to vacate the roomy and pleasant vicarage. Although members of the Culpeper family lived in the manor houses of Ockley and Wakehurst in nearby Sussex, Mary decided to move back to her father, the reverend William Attersoll, beneficed in Isfield, Sussex.

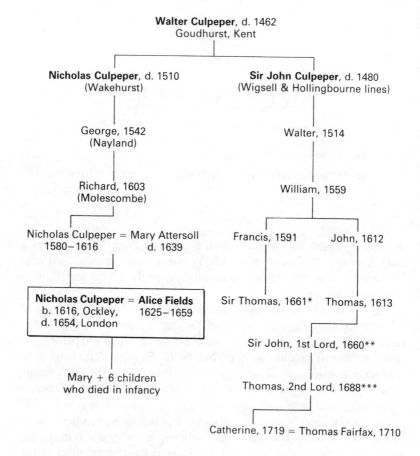

Figure 1. Culpeper Family Tree

The following text is part of the family tree:

Walter Culpeper, d. 1462
Goudhurst, Kent

Nicholas Culpeper, d. 1510
(Wakehurst)

Sir John Culpeper, d. 1480
(Wigsell & Hollingbourne lines)

George, 1542
(Nayland)

Walter, 1514

Richard, 1603
(Molescombe)

William, 1559

Nicholas Culpeper = Mary Attersoll
1580–1616   d. 1639

Francis, 1591   John, 1612

Nicholas Culpeper = Alice Fields
b. 1616, Ockley,   1625–1659
d. 1654, London

Sir Thomas, 1661*   Thomas, 1613

Sir John, 1st Lord, 1660**

Mary + 6 children
who died in infancy

Thomas, 2nd Lord, 1688***

Catherine, 1719 = Thomas Fairfax, 1710

*   of Leeds Castle, wrote 'Tract against high rate of usurie'
**   Master of the Rolls to Charles I
***   Governor of Virginia, 1677–1683

There, in the church named after the same patron saint as in Ockley, St Margaret of Antioch, the young Culpepers had been happily married, just a year earlier, on October 25th, 1615. The marriage of Attersoll's daughter to Culpeper, a gentleman divine, had been entirely to his liking. Mary was probably introduced to the promising young parson when they were invited to the Culpeper's in the not too distant manor of Wakehurst. Shortly before, the happy groom had been appointed as rector to the church in Surrey where one of his predecessors, his great-great uncle Edvard Culpeper, had already been minister in 1514. It was thought that a good family tradition had come true when Nicholas Culpeper was given his preferment.

The Culpepers were a distinguished ancient family which had been settled in the South of England for centuries. The first member mentioned in historical records appeared in the thirteenth century and was Sir Thomas de Colepeper, *'Recognitor Mangnae Assisae'*, in King John's reign. There are several lines: the Wigsell and Hollingbourne branch, the Begdebury and Aylesford Culpepers and the Culpepers of Wakehurst to which Nicholas Culpeper belonged. The coat of arms of Nicholas Culpeper is that of the Wakehurst family: Argent, a bend engrailed Gules. They all originated in Kent and later many of them settled in Sussex, Surrey and America.[4,5]

Early in their history, the Culpepers engaged in iron working and it was said that they were men of 'blood and iron'. They rose as landowners, soldiers and justices. At one time, twelve members of the family bore the honour of knighthood. Probably the most distinguised Stuart Culpeper was John Culpeper (1600–1660) of Wigsell and Hollingbourne, MP for Kent in the Long Parliament. He was made Chancellor of the Exchequer in 1642, Master of the Rolls in 1643, and was created Lord Culpeper in 1644. Being a loyal Royalist, he in 1645 accompanied Prince Charles (later Charles II) to his exile in Paris and returned to England at the Restoration in 1660. The peerage became extinct in 1725. Sir Thomas (1578–1662) was a scholar who studied at Oxford and thereafter law at the Inns of Court in London. He became famous for writing a 'Tract against Usurie'. His son, Sir Thomas the younger, continued his father's struggle for a reduction in interest rates.

No satisfactory explanation has been given for the origin of the name Culpeper or Colepeper, but it can be assumed that it was derived from a place such as Culspore in Kent. It could also be connected to an occupation such as a false pepperer, one who traded outside the guild of pepperers; or it may have been a nickname, since 'Pepper' was regarded as symbolical of giving offence. Thus Jack Straw, a contemporary rebel, was described as a 'Culpeper' or mischief maker.[6] Nicholas Culpeper belonged to the Wakehurst branch of the family. Wakehurst Place was an old rich estate in the Wealden Woodlands with iron ore and a seemingly limitless supply of wood, the basis of the Sussex iron industry. Outside the manor house were 'hammer ponds', which provided a head of water to drive the hammers and bellows for the furnaces and forgery. The original Wakehursts probably held the estate from the early part of the twelfth century until the line ended in 1454 with two girls, Margaret and Elizabeth. Placed in the charge of Sir John Culpeper of Bedgebury, they were abducted in 1463 by his brothers Richard and Nicholas who 'with force and arms riotously agense the Kynges peace, arrayed in the manner of warre at Goudhurst toke and carried them away . . . the seide Margarete and Elizabeth at the tyme of their takyng away makyng grete and pittious lamentacion and wepyng'. The 'lamentacion and wepyng' did not, however, appear to have lasted very long, as both couples were married very speedily and, when the furore had died down, lived happily together at Wakehurst Place for another fifty years. The first to die was Margaret, in 1509; Elizabeth, the last, was still alive in 1517. Richard and Margaret had no children, but Nicholas and Elizabeth had eighteen, ten sons and eight daughters, all on display on a brass plate in Ardingly church.[4,7] The beautiful Elizabethan manor house was built in 1590 by Sir Edward Culpeper and the estate remained in the Culpeper family for over 200 years until it was sold off in 1717 to pay for gambling debts. Today Wakehurst Place is an extension of Kew Gardens with a magnificent collection of rare trees and flowering shrubs[7,8] – and behind an old walled enclosure is a fragrant herb garden, which really should be dedicated to the memory of its famous ancestor, Nicholas Culpeper!

2
Youth in Sussex

These bells are like the powers of my soul;
Their clappers to the passions of my mind:
O Lord ! If thy poor child might have his will,
And might his meaning freely to him tell;
He never of his musick has his fill,
There's nothing like thy ding dong bell.

John Bunyan, 1628–1688.

The youthful years of Nicholas Culpeper's life were filled with the
sound of church bells, and services with long hours in the pew of
his grandfather William Attersoll's church, St Margaret's, in Isfield,
Sussex. The vicarage of Isfield belonged to the thaneship of the
Shurley family who lived in the nearby Tudor house, Isfield Place.
They had been given the right of presentation some time before
1527.[1,2] This meant the right of the benefactor to appoint priests
and receive tithes. The income was used to pay for the vicar, to
maintain the church and to support in hospitality to the poor.

In 1599, during the reign of Queen Elizabeth I, William Attersoll
had been appointed rector of the parish of St. Margaret's, Isfield by
the local squire and landowner Sir John Shurley. When Attersoll was
selected, he had the reputation of a scholar, with two degrees from
Cambridge. This obviously impressed John Shurley, who wanted a
learned man in his pulpit, a preacher who could bring some culture
to his parish. John Shurley might have liked the image of being a
sponsor of science, something which would be valued and perhaps
envied by his peers of the local gentry. Moreover, he wanted a
learned teacher for his nine children. Attersoll was a serious man,
more interested in books and the writing of theological treatises
than in the edification of his parishoners. He wrote many theological
books and was considered an important scholar of his time. Attersoll

was not popular with his parishoners, because he did not socialise with them, and was not an eloquent and captivating preacher like his predecessor, the reverend William Bishoppe. Attersoll had higher aspirations for his living and his surroundings; he always thought that he deserved a better place. He complained about the 'poor living and poor cottage'.[1]

In Isfield he had no intellectual intercourse with learned colleagues, as in Cambridge where he lived before. There were difficulties in getting the latest books from London, a much too small vicarage for his large family and now his daughter was back with his grandson! Attersoll was aloof and demanding in his way of life. He had six children from his first wife, Anne, who died in 1624. Five months later he married Mary Parris, the widow of his parish clerk.[3]

As mistress of the house, Anne Attersoll had a difficult and arduous task looking after the big household, to feed, clean, nurse and plan for the future. She did not have much help from her husband, who after his duties as a priest and teacher always retired to his study and his books. Her daughter, Mary, was of course a good help.

The vicarage, now called Rocks Farm, was a building of stone with a tiled roof, on a slight mound not far from the church, overlooking the meadows down to the river Ouse. On the bottom floor, on the left side of the entrance was the vicar's office and study with the parlour to the right, and the kitchen, buttery, still room and larder in the back. Around the walls were large open fire places with ornamental, locally cast-iron firebacks to protect the brickwork where the fire was hottest. In front of these were placed pairs of andirons, fire forks and spit irons. In the kitchen the andirons supported roasting-spits and on the side-boards were pewter vessels and plates, brass-pots and pans. The stone floor was covered with fresh rush-mats. Upstairs, in the bedrooms, there were beds of wood with a headpiece and canopy. These huge beds had comfortable feather-beddings with blankets and a head-sheet. Side curtains could be drawn at night. In addition to the big beds, there were a number of small, low truckle-beds which could be pushed out of the way in the day-time.

Next to the vicarage were two outhouses where the brewing, churning and slaughtering was done. In these low houses most of the servants also had their quarters. There was also a barn and stable combined in one building where horses, cows and pigs were kept. The house was sourrounded by a large herb and fruit garden. The cultivation of herbs and flowers had received great impetus since Queen Elizabeth's day. This revival was due in part to the publication of Gerard's *Herbal* in 1596, the text used by the educated and well-to-do. But in addition there were also herbals for the common men like William Turner's *Herball* of 1568 or William Langham's *Garden of Health* which appeared in 1597. It was a special privilege for the parson Attersoll to have a dovecot with a large number of pigeons always flying around the house. The pigeons were good company and a welcome source of fresh meat in the winter months when other meat and fish was salted.[4,5]

The outhouses of the vicarage were not very big because the glebe, or the portion of land assigned to the clergyman in Isfield, was rather limited. Attersoll depended for many of his needs on supplies from the big tithe-farm of the Shurley's manor house. That suited Attersol fine, because manual labour and earthly enterprises did not interest him; he was a very learned man utterly devoted to his books, the word of God and theological teachings. His study was a sacred place in the vicarage. Nobody was allowed to just run in and out. One had to knock and wait one's time. When the oaken door was opened one entered a different world: a smell of burning rush candles mixed with the undescribable fumes from old parchment and gall-nut ink. Along the walls were rows of books of all sizes stacked up to the ceiling. The big oaken table was covered with papers and books bound in vellum. Above the mantle piece glittered a silver cross. This room also contained an unusual adornment: a precious persian carpet near the chest, a gift from Sir Antony Sherley of Wiston, Sussex, a relative of Sir John Shurley. Sir Antony had been in Arabia and Persia and was a friend of Shah Abbas from whom he had received tents and carpets.[6]

Through instruction from his grandmother, and contemporary herbals such as Gerard's, Nicholas learned to recognise medicinal plants and how they were prepared and used. Already as a boy young Nicholas was interested in herbs and medicines and realised early the healing power of local plants. He loved the smells of gilliflower, Frankford roses and basil. From Culpeper's *Herbal* we know that young Nicholas was familiar with the native names of plants and flowers as they were used in Sussex. About Heart's-Ease he says: 'In Sussex we call them pansies' and the gooseberry bush in Sussex is called: 'Dew-berry bush'.[7]

Knowledge about recipes and home-cures was usually inherited from mother to daughter and kept as a valuable 'secret'. For the educated classes books such as the anonymous *Closet for ladies and Gentlewomen*, printed in 1608, were available. This included 'divers soveraigne medicines and salves for sundry diseases'. Then there was of course also Gervase Markham's famous *Countrey Contentments* which had appeared in 1615. The second part of this work was *The English House Wife* with chapters on 'Physicke, Cookery, banqueting-stuff, distillations, etc'.[8,9]

Women in the house were particularly well skilled in the art of 'simpling' and preparing medicines, a simple being a medicinal herb or medicine obtained from one herb. It was so called because each plant was supposed to possess its particular virtue, and therefore to constitute a simple remedy. Nicholas often followed his mother and grandmother to the garden and fields to pick herbs for the concoction and distillation of medicines, syrups and other 'secrets'. He was interested in these remedies since in 'The London Dispensatory' he mentions purslain: 'I remember since I was a child that it is admirable for one that hath his teeth on edge by eating sour apples.' What he means by this he explains in his *Herbal* that 'It is good for mouth and gums that are swoln and to fasten loose teeth.' In another place he says: 'Flowers are but seldom preserved; I never saw any that I remember, save cowslip flowers and that was great fashion in Sussex when I was a boy.'[10]

In those days outside the cathedral cities hardly any licensed physicians were to be found, so people had to rely either on itinerant practitioners, and cunning folk such as 'smiths, weavers, and women'. The nearest medical authority to be found was probably the town apothecary-cum-surgeon in Lewes. Often clerics or their wives were consulted for medical help. This applied to mistress Anne Attersoll who probably was an experienced healer, and from comments in Culpeper's translation of the *London Dispensatory*, we hear that young Nicholas was familiar with the names of diseases as used in Sussex. Of the plaster of Melilot he says: 'It is special good for those swellings vulgarly in London called felons, in Sussex andicoms.'[10]

The church, St Margaret's of Antioch lies on the slope down where the rivers Ouse and Uck meet, near the old Roman road leading from New Haven to London. The church had a low tower in the west, a narrow nave for the congregation and a wider chancel for the altar and the ministrations of the priest. On the north wall of the chancel was the beautiful Easter Sepulchre. Connected with the east end of the nave was the Shurley chapel, the private chantry of the endower with the tombs of John and Thomas Shurley and the squire stalls. Here the members of the Shurley family celebrated mass sitting in their oak pews and looking through a small opening in the wall, a squint, to the chancel and with the view of the Easter Sepulchre. At the time of the church service the parishioners would assemble outside the bell tower and then walk in, the men on the right and the women on the left side.[11]

Nicholas did not enjoy the obligatory long services with prayers, long sermons and particularly when his black-robed grandfather climbed into the pulpit and started his admonitions about vices and virtues and the doctrines of the church. Sometimes he thought of his own father, whom he had never seen. He could not possibly have been so boring and hard. His mother sometimes said that he had been a handsome man of gentle birth and well lettered not only in holy things but in all matters.

In church he really only enjoyed singing, and was a member of the choir singing hymns. Later he relates: 'I would willingly write a word or two to musitians, whose faculty and worthy science I exceedingly delight in. Narrowness of the windpipe is the cause of a shrill voice, and that's the reason women and boys whose windpipe is narrow, sing a treble best, and because the windpipe even in some of those is narrower than others, some of them are able to sing higher than others, even above E-la.'[12]

Nicholas' mind was always elsewhere, outside near the stables of the manor or the small riverboats on the Ouse. Youthful activities were often centered around the always attractive water were boys could fish, boat and swim. The river Ouse rises at the Wealden village of Ardingly and is fed by several small streams such as one from Uckfield and later pierces the gap in the chalk at Lewes down to the Channel. The river invited anglers since it was full of trout, chub, dace and salmon.

Some years in winter flooded fields near the confluence of the Ouse and Uck froze, transforming them into an icy pond which attracted the youth to try their luck skidding on the treacherous surface. In wet springs the waters of the Ouse and Uck often rose above their banks transforming the peaceful stretches of meadowland into a foggy sea of water with the fool'-caps shingled spire of the church rising from its slightly higher grounds. At this time it could be difficult to reach the church dry-footed so wagons had to be used for those which could not ride. During these flood times

a number of youngsters died by drowning, mostly in springtime
when they dared boat rides in small craft. (From church records
in St Margaret's we know that some youngsters were buried; after
their name there is the entry, 'drowned'.)

In winter and at Christmas time St Margaret's was lit by candles,
set in magnificent brass candelabra hung from the roof and on staves
placed in sockets at the bench ends. Outside the church, torches
burned and illuminated the walls with flickering lights.[13] On the
way from the church to the vicarage Nicholas had to pass through
the big meadows and when the lights of the church disappeared
the firmament shone bright on cloudless nights. Little Nicholas may
have looked up and thought of his father, and of his friends who had
died in the floods. Were they looking at him from above – because
surely they must be in heaven, and what did they want to tell him
when he saw the falling stars, and could they reveal events of life?
Were not stars the eyes of heaven?

In 1625 there were especially many shooting stars. Nicholas was
frightened, and ran to his grandfather and told him about it. That
was at a time when news had reached Isfield that the Black Death, or
plague, raged in London. Soon rumours were heard that Robert, the
brother of Sir John Shurley, had died in the City. William Attersoll,
as the official representative of the church and the King, received a
notice about the plague to be posted and announced in the church.
At the same time he also received from his bookseller in London
a pamphlet of how to combat the disease. This included general
recommendations to keep houses, yards, streets and channels clean
from standing puddles, dung hills and corrupt moistures: 'to suffer
no dogs nor cats to come into the houses and to fumigate rooms
with frankincense, likewise to perfume apparell with juniper.' It also
contained 59 receipts for preservatives against the plague containing
cloves, walnuts, cinnamon, nutmeg, wormwood, 'pestilent-wort'
and numerous other herbs.[14] When Attersoll showed this tract to
his grandson he became very interested. Attersoll said that if such
a multitude of ingredients were recommended for the same ailment,
none of them could really be effective, otherwise there was no need
for this vast compilation. Nicholas took this to his heart and thought
of ways to predict and prevent the pestilence.

Young Nicholas was a contemplative child who always asked
the question 'why'. Why did he not see his father like all the
other children in the village? Why did grandmother collect all the
flowers and dry them? He liked to watch the stars at night, but

what happened with them during the day? Did they go to sleep? Grandfather William's clocks were Nicholas' first encounter with the world of the supernatural.

Nicholas had always been fascinated with the sun-dial on the south side of St Margaret's. Early on he realised that the moving shadow of the sun had a great power over everybody in the village. It prompted the start of service and the church ales. Therefore the sun ruled his grandfather, the lord of the manor and everybody else in Isfield village. Could the moon cast a shadow at night and could it tell the time like the sun? One evening he secretly climbed down the stairs from the bedroom, to look at the moon in the open. He erected a stick in the courtyard and saw the shadow move on the ground. Did it tell the time like the sun or did it foretell something else?

He was convinced that the sun and stars also ruled the little oval verge watch in gilt bronze and the lantern clock of his grandfather. The verge watch looked like an egg. It showed not only the time in Roman numerals on a ring dial inside the cover but also reproduced the movement of the solar system with planets and all. So watching the heavens gave way to watching of the hands on a dial. How could the moving hands on the dial show the time on a cloudy day and at night? Was there a little sun inside the watch? Maybe he could tell by feeling if it was warm? Nicholas was not allowed to touch the precious and mysterious piece. What was inside? One day, when Nicholas was alone in the house he went to grandfather's study, and carefully took the watch out of its box. It felt cold, not hot at all, so there could not be a little burning sun inside. Was it a cool moon?

By pressing with his fingers on a little rim he heard a clicking sound and a lid on the backside opened. Looking inside increased the mystery: it was a glittering maze of shining tiny wheels and moving parts. So there was light and life inside! Nicholas was frightened, closed the lid and put the miracle watch back into its case. Later he asked grandfather who told him that the life and movement of the timepiece simply had to do with winding it with a key! He said that this was a very precious thing made by Edmund Gilpin in London and presented to him by Sir Henry Fenshaw. Nicholas could not believe that this was the whole truth.

Young Nic (as he was known locally) soon developed into an agile young man, a spitfire in temper and passions. He received his first schooling together with the Shurley children in the manor house; his grandfather acted as tutor. There for the first time he met the beautiful Judith Rivers. Her brother James had married Charity Shurley on July 22nd 1624.[3]

When he was ten his mother decided that he should attend the well-known grammar school at Lewes, established in 1248. 'Nicholas was educated at a Free-School in Sussex, at the cost and charges of his mother.'[15] We have reason to believe that it was the same which was chosen for John Evelyn instead of Eton. When John Evelyn in 1630 attended the 'Free School at Southover' in Lewes, Nicholas must already have been a pupil.[16] The school enjoyed a good reputation, since it was preferred to Eton by the father of John Evelyn, the famous diarist, who was probably a schoolmate with Culpeper.

In the summer of 1628, when Nicholas was 12 years old, his mother wanted to make a trip to London to see her sister Elizabeth in Holborn.[17] Nicholas nagged and nagged to be taken with her and finally she agreed but not without some scornful comments from grandfather William. They took a coach and reached the George Inn in Southwark, London, late in the evening. The next morning when they approached the Southwark gate of London Bridge, Nicholas noted with horror a large number of human heads spiked on poles on Traitor's Tower, the entry of the narrow bridge gate. One was still fresh with blood dripping down the pole. Mary had to explain that these were the heads of illdoers and beastly criminals who had been beheaded in the Tower on the other side of the river. (Thomas Culpeper's head had been on display here in 1542. Thomas, a relative of Nicholas, was beheaded together with his cousin, Cathrine Howard, Henry VIII's unfaithful wife.) Entering the bridge road was like going through a gate of a world of fancy: signs of numerous shops of needlemakers, haberdashers, glovemakers, booksellers, and a chapel. The road was crowded with carts and passers by. Strange smells and shouts resounded between the dark arches. It was a truly frightening and at the same time tempting experience. Little Nicholas was full of questions, and his mother told him about famous craftsmen and artisans of the bridge such as Hans Holbein, the German painter who once maintained a workshop there and Sir William Hewet the wealthy clockmaker and Lord Mayor of London. Hewet's daughter once fell out of a window into the Thames and the young apprentice John Osborne gallantly leaped into the river and brought out the child hail and healthy. Sir William was very grateful to John who later married the young lass.[18]

On their way back to Isfield they again passed the bridge and went to the George Inn from where their Sussex coach was going to start its journey. When they arrived in the morning the innkeeper said that the wheels of the coach had broken and he could not tell when the next coach would go. 'Maybe to-morrow, maybe after to-morrow. But take your time and rest with us, I will give you an excellent room on the second floor, close to the gallery with a good view over the courtyard.' The Ashwill company had just arrived to set up the play *The Merry Wives of Windsor* by the late William Shakespeare in the nearby Globe theatre. Nicholas was allowed to watch the performance in the afternoon. He loved it and cried out laughing at the fat John Falstaff and the stupid doctor Caius, the French physician who did not speak proper English.

When Nicholas was 13 years of age he became an avid reader, and his grandfather's library provided him with ample material: books of all kinds and sizes, broadsheets and prints, and of course Bibles in English, Greek and Latin, and prayer books. Young Nicholas was particularly attracted to the mysteries of life and the universe. Already when he was ten he started reading astrological and medical texts such as almanacs and Sir Christopher Heydon's *A Defence of Judicial Astrology*.

His interest was not so much in religious matters but rather he looked for anything that had to do with natural sciences, medicine and astrology. He was very fond of the *New Herball* by William Turner which contained illustrations of plants and described their virtues. Old Attersoll was proud of it and said:

'This is a book of a great man who defended the true religion against popery. He had to leave England during Queen Mary's reign but returned when our great Queen Elizabeth ascended the throne.'
'What was your beloved queen like?' asked Nicholas. 'She was a defender of our English faith, she was a learned lady and liked flowers and art,' and he whispered; 'she was not like the present Scottish upstart. There will never be anybody like her.'

One day he found a tiny little book entitled: *Anatomie of Man's Body*, written by the Barber Surgeon to King Henry the VIII, Thomas Vicary.[19] In the introduction it reads: 'And albeit this treatise be small in volume, yet in commoditie it is great and profitable.'

Nicholas took a quick look, saw the frightening picture of a
human skeleton and decided that this was for him. He grabbed
the book, hid it under his shirt and ran away to the barn so that
he would not be disturbed reading it. He knew that his grandfather
did not like him reading everything that was on the shelf. He only
encouraged him to read the Bible and some educational scripts.
When he arrived at the barn he climbed the hayloft and opened
the big gates on the gavel to let the sunshine in. He leafed through
the pages and decided to start where it said 'The hanches and their
parts.' For he was most interested to learn something about the
secrets of the private parts and the mysteries of reproduction. He
keenly began reading:

> And forasmuch as it has pleased almightie God to give the
> knowledge of these mysteries: the embyryon is a thing in the
> mothers womb, the original thereof is the sparme of the man
> and the women. This sparme that cometh both of men and
> woman, is made and gathered of the most best and purest
> drops, of blood in all the body, and by the labor and chasing
> of the testikles or stones. And in man it is hotte, white and
> thick and the womens sparme has contrarie qualities, for the
> womens sparme is thinner, colder and feebler. And as some
> authors, hold opinion, when this matter is gathered into the
> right side of the matrix, then it happeneth a male kinde, and
> likewise on the left a female. And further it is to be noted,
> that as like the renet of the cheese hath by himself the way and
> virtue of working, so has the milk by waye of suffering: and as
> the way and milk make the cheese, so doth the sparme of man
> and women by the virtue of kindly heat make the generation
> of embryon.

And then he went on looking for more secret information as he
read:

> The parts proceeding outwardly are didimus, peritoneum, the
> yarde and testikles. And first shall be spoken of the yarde,
> or of mans generative members, which place is from the
> coddes unto the fundament. The yarde is an official member,
> and the tyller of mans generation, compound and made of
> skinne, brawnes, tendons, veynes, arteirs, senews and great
> ligaments: and it has in it two passages, of principle issues,

that is to say one for the sparme and one for the urin. And as the philosophers say, the quantitie of the yard is five or six ynches, with measurable bignes proportioned to the quantitie of the matrix. This member hath, as sayth Avincen, three holes, through one passeth insencible polissions and wynde, that causeth the yard to rise, the other two holes be declared before. Also the yard has a skinne, and about the head thereof it is double, and that man call preputium and this skinne is movable, for through this consecration the spermatike matter is the better and sooner gathered together, and sooner cast for forth from the testicles: for by him is hade more delectation in the doing. The coddes, is a compound member. This purse was ordained for the custodie and comfort of the testicles and other spermatic vessels. The testikles or stones are two, made of glandulus fleshe or cornelly fleshe. And further more through the didimus comest to the testikles from the brayne, senowes and from the heart arteirs, and from the lyver veynes, bringing onto them both feeling and steering, lyfe and spirite, and nutrimental blood, and the most purest blood of al other members of the body, whereof is made the sparme by the labour of the testikles, the which is put forth in due tyme, as before rehearsed.

After reading this he was also greatly perplexed and when he went to bed he contemplated the strange issue of a baby being conceived in his mother's womb like a cheese. 'A smelly cheese?!' There must be more mystery to this and he was eager to find out for himself one day. He did, and later devoted two sections and ten chapters in his *Directory for Midwives* (1651) to the organs of procreation. The influence of Vicary's old text (1577) is clearly discernible.

Who influenced Culpeper's personality and thinking? One of them certainly was his grandfather, William Attersoll. Culpeper undoubtedly had a love-hate relationship with him. He admired and inherited his great wit and easy pen but he disliked his stern authoritarian character, the way he wanted to shape him to become a minister, his attitude towards smoking and his dislike of the extraordinary which interested Nicholas so much.

William Attersoll was the typical country parson, a sober, scholarly and poetic minister and the toady of his squire. Village life revolved around him and the lord of the manor. Absorbed by his books had become aloof, neglected his duties as a friend of his people, and did not participate in Whitsun ales, harvest festivities, All Hallow Evening and Christmas Mummings. Attersoll was a man greatly learned in classical lore. Not only did he know the Bible from beginning to the end but he also had a wonderful recollection of many Greek and Latin authors, like the astrological canon *tetrabiblos* of Ptolemy. He was a strange character, a famous author of his time, but totally ignorant of human nature and the ways of the world. He wrote many volumes on Christian dogma and moral teachings.

Why was he like that? Set a refined and scholarly man down in a little country parish with no society but simple farmers and a country squire, pigs, cows and sheep, with little chance of mixing with people of like intellect and learning and it would be remarkable if he had not developed some signs of eccentricity. Nicholas feared and admired him and was certainly without wanting influenced by the rector of Isfield, his grandfather and father-figure.

Grandfather Attersoll exerted great influence on the future astrological physician. In his writings he mentions the influence of 'divers signs' on the human being, 'some are naturell, as the clouds be the signs of raine, the redness of the skye in the evening of fair weather. Some are miraculous such as shall be in the sun and moon, in the stares'.[20] He spoke of himself as a prophet: 'A prophet is not without honour safe in his own country and among his own kinne, and his own house'; he considered himself the mediator of 'Physick against Famine, or a soveraigne preservative against all distrustfull thoughts and cares touching the things of this life, prescribed and administered by the best physicians of sole and body, Christ Jesus'.[21]

Attersoll, who saw his mission as educating his flock, spoke about 'the necessary duty of teaching'. Puritan preachers were terrible sinners in the matter of the length of their sermons, preaching being the essential part of the service, far more important than worshipping and praying to God. The sermon usually should not exceed one hour, and in order to remind the preacher of the flight of time the hourglass had become a constant addition to the 17th-century pulpit. But its restraining influence was not always exercised and some parsons, like Attersoll delighted in turning the glass. His sermons where terribly long and demanding and it happened that the congregation saw the sand run out twice during a sermon.

On one occasion when preaching against drunkenness, he said: 'If we had no law and ordinances, ale houses would be fuller stuffed and thronged than our church . . . '[20] Nicholas, whose attendance at Sunday sermons was compulsory, began to yawn at the end of a single glass. Attersoll, however, not to be silenced by a yawn, turned his time-keeper and desired his congregation to be patient a while longer, for he had much more to say about the vice of alcohol; 'therefore', he added, 'my friends and brethren, we will have another glass' and then he went on with his accusation of sinners.

3
Cambridge and Youthful Protest

I am a master of myself, as of the Universe;
I am and wish to be.

Pierre Corneille, 1606–1684

In the 17th century, university life started early. Francis Bacon was sent to Trinity College when he was thirteen and John Milton to Christ's at sixteen. In 1632, at the age of sixteen, Nicholas Culpeper started his studies at Cambridge.

His grandfather and mother had decided that he should follow in the footsteps of his father and become a minister. They made the necessary arrangements for him to go up to his old *Alma Mater*, where both his father and grand-father had started their own studies.[1] (It is not known, however, with any certainty which College he was admitted to. If it was Christ College he could have met John Milton just as he was leaving after having received his Masters of Art degree *cum laude*. It could also have been Caius College, which was noted for medicine.)

Cambridge University was the stronghold of protestantism and later puritanism. The famous Erasmus of Rotterdam had taught there and Queen Elizabeth favoured Cambridge more than Oxford. Culpeper's grandfather, the puritan reverend William Attersoll, spent a long time in Cambridge where he studied at Jesus College, Clare Hall and Peterhouse before he was appointed to the living in Isfield in 1599. It is therefore not surprising that Cambridge was also chosen for Nicholas to study.

As the son of a Gentleman, young Nicholas entered as a fellow-commoner and not as a sizar or pensioner (the sizar was a position which enabled poorer boys to obtain a university education in

18

exchange for services in the College and the pensioner was one who obtained a scholarship). Most fellow-commoners usually belonged to two main categories: they were either sons of the aristocracy and did not really come for serious studies but to obtain the polish of higher education, or they studied for holy orders and became parish priests. Culpeper was supposed to belong to the latter category but he himself was of a different opinion.

In Cambridge, the old tradition which regarded Latin as the hallmark of educated man was still unchallanged. A freshman had to be competent in Latin, since most teachers and textbooks were in that language. Every boy who completed grammar school had worked at Latin for seven years. In addition, Nicholas had had a good introduction to Greek while in Lewes. There is good reason to believe that Culpeper had the same opinion about the curriculum offered in Cambridge as John Milton who said that students were fed 'with nothing else but the scragged and thorny lectures of monkish and miserable sophistry'.[2]

His grandfather was determined that Culpeper should devote himself to divinity, but the boy preferred medicine. To begin with, the studies were essentially identical and consisted mainly of the classical languages, Latin and Greek. He was bored by the method of teaching which involved mostly translations of classical authors such as Plato into Latin and Cicero into Greek, and he certainly would have preferred to study medicine full time. But he probably often sneaked out from these exercises to more stimulating lectures about *materia medica* and anatomy.

The study of medicine was difficult to pursue, and he met resistance from his mother and grandfather. It was lengthy, and teachings in physick (medicine) and anatomy were not so well developed in England as on the continent. Most of the more eminent contemporary physicians of his time like Harvey and Sydenham had studied abroad. Padua, Montpellier, Paris and Leyden were the centres of medical teaching. Usually after finishing a basic degree at Oxford or Cambridge to become proficient in classical languages students of medicine went abroad to get an MD degree from one of these acknowledged universities. In addition, sons of wealthy parents went on a grand tour of Europe to polish their general knowledge and to study modern languages like French.

The notable physician Francis Glisson (1597–1677) was an exception. It is possible that Culpeper met him just before Glisson took his MD degree at Caius College, Cambridge, in 1634. Glisson later became Regius Professor of Physick at the same university. He was one of the founders of the Royal Society and was elected president of the College of Physicians. In 1651 Culpeper translated his famous 'Tractatus de Rachitide' and in 1654 the 'Anatomia hepatis'.

When he came to Cambridge the centre of the town was not unlike its modern self. With minor alterations the river Cam was on its present course, the chief bridges had been built and the main streets had taken their form. The original thirteen colleges were already established. Each college had its own tennis court and several had bowling-greens and fish ponds. The young students usually were not given much ready cash. Responsible for the costs of studies were the tutors, who were paid for everything that could be considered an ordinary requirement for a student: teaching fees, books, food, housing and even clothes. There were no college clubs, and very few opportunities of spending money in ways not forbidden by academic statutes.[3] But young Nicholas spent lavishly on extracurricular activities. 'His mother spent four hundred pounds on her said son, for his diet, schooling, and being at the university of Cambridge.'[4]

His stay at Cambridge was not for long. He did not take his compulsory studies seriously and never graduated, although it was his highest ambition to become a physician. He was often found in taverns of the town and engaged in sports like tennis and bowling.

He went up to Cambridge with the high expectation of a young gentleman who wanted to enjoy life. At the University, besides formal learning, many useful contacts for a successful life could be made. All sons of Britain's important families went to Oxford or Cambridge before embarking on their professional careers. To obtain the fashionable polish of society was just as important as to sit for a degree. Therefore his mother did not spare money to enable Nicholas to benefit as much as possible from all aspects of College life.

Young Nicholas was not looking forward to studying theology but he was anxious to be introduced to all the leisure activities like fencing, bowling, bear and bull-baiting and tennis. These sports had become fashionable and an essential part of liberal education and were frequently practised despite the fact that some had been banned by the Elizabethan Statutes at Cambridge. The statutes, however, were consistently disregarded and certain illegal activities like bear and bull-baiting were carried out in the nearby town of Chesterton or in the Gogmagog Hills. One of the few games that was permitted was football, but it was prescribed that it should only be played within the college courts or gardens and no matches should ever be played outside the college. 'Fote bale' was freely indulged in, and matches with outsiders were carried on, all statutes to the contrary notwithstanding.[3]

To have an idea of what his life might have been like, listen to John Earle's tale of 1628:

> A mere young gentleman of the university is one that comes there to wear a gown, and to say hereafter, he has been at the university. His father sent him thither because he heard there were the best fencing and dancing schools; from these he has his education, from his tutor the oversight. The first element of his knowledge is to be shown the colleges, and initiated in a tavern by the way, which hereafter he will learn of himself. The two marks of his seniority is the bare velvet of his gown and his proficiency at tennis, where when he can once play at set he is a freshman no more. His study has commonly handsome shelves, his books neat silk strings, which he shews his father's man, and is loth to untie or take down for fear of misplacing. Upon foul days for recreation he retires thither, and looks over the pretty book his tutor reads to him, which is commonly some short history, or a piece of Euphormio; for which his tutor gives him money to spend next day.[5]

While in Cambridge, Culpeper had picked up the habit of smoking and 'drinking' tobacco. The rich young gallant carried his apparatus about with him, tobacco-box, ladle, priming iron, and pipes. Smoking certainly was a fashionable accomplishment. When the students escaped from the strict discipline and the narrow quandrangle of their college they competed with each other in the performance of every possible vice. Smoking was one of them. There were indeed even 'schools', on the analogy of fencing and dancing schools, where the fashionable art of smoking was taught.

Cambridge was surrounded by a lot of water and deep fens and boggy ground, not very attractive and unhealthy. The waters were infested with mosquitoes, insects which transmitted malaria. Culpeper had experience of this, and wrote about 'tertian or quartan agues', the willow-herb, 'the smoke hereof being burned driveth away flyes and gnats which used in the night-time to molest inhabitants near marshes and in the fenney countries'.[6] But the

environment also had special attractions. One of the chief recrea-
tions of Cambridge students was the river Cam and its continuation,
the Great Ouse. The Cam was just outside the windows of the
colleges and very inviting for water sports. Peterhouse College,
located in the south of Cambridge near Trumpington Gate, was
quite near the mill pool of the river Cam, an excellent facility for
swimming and fishing. Swimming had been the rage after Everard
Digby in 1587 published his delightfully illustrated treatise *'De arte
natandi'* or: 'The art of swimming'. In 1595, translated into English,
it became very popular with students. Every conceivable trick and
posture in swimming and diving was described. Digby was a fellow
of St John's College, an odd character who 'was in the habit of
blowing a horn and hallooing in the college during the daytime,
and repeatedly spoke of the master to the scholars with the greatest
disrespect'. Because of his undisciplined manners he was expelled
from Cambridge.[7] (Everard the swimmer should not be confused
with Sir Everard Digby, the conspirator of the Gunpowder plot.)

Swimming in Cambridge had become a very popular sport, so
much so that repeated casualties had occurred among the young
and unexperienced country squires who plunged into the waters,
particularly near Grandchester. This is evident from the parish
register since there are frequent entries about several students who
drowned. Swimming was therefore prohibited by the time Culpeper
arrived on the scene. But this did not prevent the adventerous
boy from showing off in front of his friends; on the contrary,
forbidden fruit was even more to his liking, moreover, he was
well experienced in this sport from his previous aquatic exercises
in the Sussex Ouse.

While in Cambridge he kept up contact with his childhood
sweetheart Judith Rivers. They had known each other as children,
and met for the first time at the wedding of her brother, James Rivers
and Charity, the daughter of Sir John Shurley, in Isfield Place, the
manor house of the Shurleys. It was on July 22, 1624 when Nicholas
was barely eight and Judith nine. Thereafter Judith was a frequent
guest in Isfield where she again met young Nicholas.[8,9]

When Nicholas was invited to Isfield Place, she had caught his
eye, a somewhat shy but temperamental girl who quickly responded
to his approaches in a way that excited him. She pretended not to
understand his sentiments and played hide and seek. She spoke
more to his Wakehurst cousin, William, than to him and showed
herself briefly only to disappear in the cavernous manor house. She

liked to ride and, although he was not much of a horseman, he tried to follow her.

When Nicholas was a boarder at the Grammar school in Lewes, James Rivers moved to nearby Hamsey. Nicholas was a frequent guest and again met Judith.[10] These meetings, hardly noticed by anybody, were considered innocent plays and not until later, when again at Isfield, did Nicholas reveal the secrets of his heart. It was then that they were to be parted forever: Nicholas sent away to Cambridge and Judith out of reach to Lewes.

Joining the University at Cambridge was a painful separation and when he wrote her longing letters, she waited and did not immediately reply. But when in the end she responded to his approaches, she was wholeheartedly involved and they agreed to secret meetings; their highest wish was to be united in marriage. It was during his time in Cambridge that Culpeper made the fateful decision to elope with Judith Rivers.

The choice of a suitable partner, which was often done very early, lay entirely with the parents and many important matters had to be considered. By carefully planned alliances a nobleman hoped to widen his influence and estate. Therefore property, social position, religion and politics were more important than personal inclination.[11] The fatherless Nicholas Culpeper although of a good family, but without prospect of a considerable inheritance, certainly was not a good match for the Rivers' daughter who had a big dowry.

Nicholas was frustrated and disappointed with his studies in Cambridge. He was not allowed to study medicine but forced to prepare himself for a post in the Church. Archbishop Laud wanted to impose strict rules of moral conduct and catholic rituals of worship. What was his future? He then made the fateful decision to start a life of his own, away from the established society.

When it became clear that they could not be married with Judith's parents consent they made the extraordinary decision to elope and try to get married in secret. Now things happened quickly. The plan was that they would be secretly married and temporarily settle in the Netherlands, while awaiting a reconciliation with their parents. At the beginning of summer it was decided that they should meet near Lewes to be secretly married by Nicholas' friend from Cambridge, the young parson at Firle. Nicholas extracted more money from his weak mother, pretending that he needed cash for books and new clothes. Judith collected her valuable

inherited jewellery and made for the secret meeting place with
her servant.

When Nicholas approached Lewes the sky was covered with
thunderclouds and looked like a black furnace above the peaks of
the trees which were sometimes outskined by lightning. He was
excited and could not wait to see his sweetheart. We are told the
following, horrible details by his amanuensis, Mr. William Ryves:

> One of the first diversions that he had amongst some other
> small transactions and changes, none of his life proving more
> unfortunate, was, that he had engaged himself in the love of
> a beautiful lady; I shall not name her for some reasons; her
> father was reported to be one of the noblest and wealthiest
> in Sussex. This fair lady after many generous treatments, as
> Mr. Culpeper might clearly perceive, entertained the tenders
> of his service, so far as to requite him with her entire and
> sincere affections; and though the strictness of parents have
> often too severe eyes over their children, yet where hearts
> are once united, lovers use to break through all difficulties.
> The riches of the lady, (which might have enchanted inferior
> spirits) in respect of the vertous inclinations of her minde and
> person, had no power over him, so that like a true lover, the
> language of his eyes and his heart were the same, insomuch
> that the languishing sincerities of these suffering inamorato's,
> put them to the extremity of the determination, some way to
> set a period to their martyrdoms. Mr Culpeper having then
> supplied himself with two hundred pounds from his mother,
> during his abode at Cambridge his fair mistress and he by
> letters and otherwise, plotted secretly with the assistance of
> a Gentlewomen that waited on her, to pack up such rich
> jewels, and other neccessaries as might best appertain to a
> journey, and so secretly to make their escape near to Lewis
> in Sussex, where they intended to marry; and afterwards for a
> season to live privately till the incensed parents were pacified;
> but this happiness was denied them by the malevolence of
> Mars, and some other envious planets, as you shall find in his
> nativity. Not to vex the expectation of the reader any longer,
> but rather to epitomize so sad a story, Mr. Culpeper hastes
> from Cambridge.
>
> His mistress with those that she durst trust, were gone part
> of their way to meet him at the appointed place; but it pleased

the great disposer of terrene affairs to order it otherwise; the lady and her servants being suddenly surprized with a dreadful storme, with fearful claps of thunder, surrounded with flames of fire and flashes of lightening, with some of which Mr. Culpeper's fair mistress was so stricken, that she immediately fell down dead, exchanging of this life for a better; her marriage on earth for one in heaven. When the lady was stripped all the marks that could be found on her fair body, was only a blue spot on her right side about the breadth of ones hand.

The news of this sad accident met Mr. Culpeper as he journed towards his dead to him, but otherwise a still living saint. At the instant when this direful mischance befell him, Sir Nicholas Astey his intimate acquaintance passing by, chanced to be an eye-witness of this sad disaster, who used the best rhetorik he had to comfort him in his affliction. He took him up in his coach, and conveyed him to his mother, who not expecting then to have seen him, received him with a great deal of joy, till being so truly sensible of his sorrows; she for that cause left that county, and afterwards fell into a fit of sickness which she was never rid of till her dying day.

It is impossible to express the sorrow of so true a lover Mr. Culpeper was, the strangeness of his misfortune being enough to shake the strongest resolutions of the most established person in the world; I shall only acquaint the reader with what I have heard of his best friends, that when that he was serious even to entertain the deepest melancholy that his frailty could suffer on earth, that then he would discourse at large the sad fate of his unfortunate mistress. This lady on whom this unhappy accident fell, had two thousand pounds in personal estate, and five hundred pounds a year. The loss of his jewel which Mr. Culpeper valued above all worldly considerations, cast him in so deep a melancholy, that he left the University of Cambridge; so that it was high time for his grandfather Mr William Attersol in whose care he was, to think of some seasonable way to divert his extraordinary distemper.[12]

The death of Judith must have been a terrible blow not only to Nicholas but also to his mother and grandfather. The relationship with Judith was a shame to both families, the Rivers and Culpepers. Nicholas was devastated: he went into hiding and did not return for a long time. Mary Culpeper was deeply hurt and depressed. Grandfather William was very angry but after some time he tried to talk sense to Nicholas.

It became necessary to send him away to start a new life. It was out of the question to return to Cambridge and therefore Attersoll came up with the idea of sending him up to London to learn a useful trade. In the present situation the career as an apothecary was an appropriate choice. Nicholas always had shown an interest in all aspects of medicine both in Isfield and later in Cambridge, where he had attended lectures on Galen and Hippocrates. It had always been his ambition to become a doctor and to go abroad to study in Italy where the great advances in anatomy were being made. Mother Mary and grandfather Williams, however, always maintained that they only sent him to the University to become a minister.

When his grandfather spoke about his future and explained to him that he had to repent by doing useful work, Nicholas reflected that now, when the path to medicine had been closed, why not become an apothecary. He realised that he had sinned and that the death of Judith was a punishment from God – a punishment against his ill-doings, his empty and useless past.

The contrast beween Culpeper's extravagant style in Cambridge and the rest of his active life as we know it is striking. So much so that we have to assume that he had a radical change of mind, like Saul: 'And Saul arose from the earth and they brought him into Damascus. . . . and he was three days without sight, and neither did eat not drink . . . ' Saul's eyes were opened: 'there fell from his eyes as it had been scales, and he received sight forthwith.' So started the conversion of Saul to become Paul and in similar ways now Nicholas broke with his past and decided to go to work.

4

Mortar & Pestle

Saabean odours from the spicy shore
Of Araby the blest.

John Milton, 1608–1674

'Mr. Attersol with the advice of his friends, consulted how to dispose of Mr. Culpeper, which was to send him to London where they placed him with Mr. White, an apothecary near Temple Bar, to whom they gave with him fifty pounds; he having not been with him above a year and a half, Mr White failed, his necessities compelling him to go into Ireland with the loss of Mr. Culpepers money.'

'Culpeper, hower, did not lack good friends to stand by him in troubles. He had become acquainted with Mr. Drake, an apothecary, who had his shop in Threadneedle Street, within Bishopsgate. Culpeper was welcomed to live with his new master and another apothecary, Mr. Samuel Leadbeaters.' According to William Ryves that is what happened to his master when he came to London to become an apprentice.[1]

Why did Attersoll choose to sent his grandson to London to become an apothecary? There were probably several reasons. Attersoll was a puritan and he therefore probably shared the view of John Milton who favoured a useful education of apothecaries, architects, mariners etc. We also know from the *English Physitian* that young Nicholas had a keen interest in the medicinal herbs and flowers he saw in Isfield and Lewes. Obviously this meant that Culpeper had a liking for medicine since early childhood. University studies in Cambridge with the aim to make him a minister had been a disaster. The academic atmosphere must have been a disappointment for a young man keen to study medicine. At the time there was no 'physick garden' (like in Oxford or London) and public dissections had been suspended.[2] Moreover, young Nicholas by his extravagant lifestyle had spent most of his patrimony in these unsuccessful studies. Therefore an apprenticeship in London probably appealed to Culpeper as a solution to his dilemma.

'Nicholas Culpepper, son of Nicholas Culpepper late of Ockley in the County of Surrey, clerk in holy orders, examined and bound to Simon White for 8 years from that date.' This is the entry in the Court Book of the Apothecaries Society, *'Decimo quarto die Novembris* 1634', signed by three wardens of the Society.[3] It marks a new and decisive episode in the life of young Nicholas, who finally had come out of hiding from Isfield. It ended the period of depression and unrest after Judith's death.

After the privileged student years in Cambridge, it must have been rather difficult to adjust to the restricted existence of an apprentice in London. Particularly being a spoiled gentleman might have led to problems. City regulations stated short hair, prohibited apprentices from wearing any clothing except that provided by their masters and assessed fines for engaging in dancing or masking, for being present at tennis courts or bowling alleys, for attending cock fights or brothels, and for keeping chests or trunks without permission.[4]

We do not know much about this first period of his apprenticeship except that Nicholas was well provided for by his mother and that Simon White was not a reliable master but went bankrupt and left for Ireland. Fortunately the Apothecaries Society took its responsibility for the training of their apprentices seriously and selected another master. The entry in their Court Book reads: 'Nicholas Culpeper is turned over to Francis Drake 25 February 1636.' Mr. Drake was a young master, only 32 years of age when Culpeper joined him. He lived in Threadneedle Street. Training with Mr. Drake was much better and here he made friends with another apothecary apprentice, Samuel Leadbetter. Unfortunately for the two their master died in February of 1639 and both were: 'turned over to Mr. Higgins for the residence of his time.' Mr. Higgins was an important man, he was a warden of the Society.[3]

Training of young apothecaries not only included working for their masters but also such activities as excursions to the country-side to identify and collect medinal herbs. We know this from entries in the Apothecaries Court Book which records: 'Simpling day, 11 June 1639' and again 'Simpling day 2 July 1640' These activities were led by Mr. Thomas Johnson, assistant of the Society, and editor of the newly enlarged edition of John Gerard's famous *Herbal*. Johnson was a very important man. He had a physick garden on Snow Hill and was acquainted with the royal gardener John Tradescant and John Parkinson, apothecary to Charles I. He later participated on the Royal side in the Civil War and was killed in action.

One day Mr. Drake asked Culpeper to go down to Cheapside with horse and wagon to get some provisions and herbs from the druggist, John Robertson. While he was standing in the warehouse a young man by the name of Pieter with short blond hair and healthy red cheeks came up and asked if he could help him. Culpeper took from his pocket a paper with a list of the herbs and other compounds he required.

Culpeper noticed that his English was not perfect and he had a definite Dutch accent. When it came to ordering spermaceti oil, that precious product from the head of the sperm whale used for many medicines, young Pieter said:

'This is precious stuff obtained during ordeals which have killed many seamen. Before I came to London I was involved in getting such oil from the northern sea last year when I went on a fateful expedition to Spitsbergen with the Dutch whaling fleet to hunt for the aquatic monsters.'

'So, really, tell me what happened?'

'Yes, during that lengthy campaign in a winter camp on that remote and fearful island with ferocious white bears and wolves I nearly lost my life, not because of these creatures but scurvy, and I was one of the few survivors from the winter camp in 1634.[5] I really was in bad shape with bleedings of the gums and bloody stools. But I survived and was cured as if by a miracle. When I came back to Holland I decided never to go back to Spitsbergen. So when Mr. Robertson came to Amsterdam and offered me a position in London I gladly accepted. Now I receive most of the orders in his wharehouse and I am responsible for getting merchandise from Holland, things like blubber oil, Spermaceti, Ambergris and whalebone.'

'How were you cured, my friend?'

'Well, when we arrived at Spitsbergen in summer I had picked a supply of scurvy grass, those dainty little green leaves which creep on the ground. Our captain had advised us to collect as much as possible for the winter on the nearby hills, which we then called the "Salad Mountains". I was the only one who kept on eating it like a cow, even though the grass was frozen, bitter and course. But the others just refused to eat, they said they were not animals.'

Culpeper's face lit up when he heard the story and jumped with joy and cried:

'Thank God, heavenly father. This is another token of your divine providence. You supply us with remedies wherever we are on the globe, in the artic north or the scorching south. You lucky Pieter, praise the Lord, you are a living testimony of the law of God who givest simple medicine for all distempers anywhere on the globe. We do not have to travel far to get the right physic, all is provided for near us. In England we should take English herbs and in America American simples.'

We can assume that during his apprenticeship Culpeper learned a great deal about drugs at the same time as pursuing his private medical studies by reading modern books that had come to England from the Continent. His master probably did not object to this, and in fact, we hear that he taught him Latin in the process. As we shall see later, he probably also attended anatomy demonstrations given by the surgeons.

Culpeper must have disliked being the servant of physicians and he could be critical about their type of medicine practised, since he knew exactly what the prescriptions contained. They were chiefly empirical nostrums selected without reference to scientific principles and mostly heterogenous mixtures of substances, some of which could neutralize others. One of the most striking instances was Mithridate, which was a compound of seventy-two ingredients. Crab's eyes, snails, vipers, the urine of men and animals, calculous concretions, various portions of criminals, such as the thigh bone of a hanged man, and many other absurd remedies, extolled for different disorders.

During his apprenticeship Culpeper not only learned the art of pharmacy, but also became aware of the limitations imposed on the apothecaries. Always being a proud man, he did not like being looked down at by the physicians who enjoyed special privileges. Before the Society of Apothecaries was established as an independent body the physicians had been empowered to enter the houses of apothecaries in London, 'to search, view, and see the apothecary wares, drugs and stuff and to destroy such as they found unfit for use'.

The barbers and surgeons were restricted to their trade and were not allowed to give internally taken medicines; the physicians, however, were permitted to practice surgery. In the year 1553, the College of Physicians obtained a new act, in which it is stated that: 'Four censors, or any three of them, shall have authority to examine, survey, govern, correct, and punish all singular physicians and practisers in the faculty of physic, apothecaries, druggists, distillers, and sellers of waters and oils, and preparers of chemical medicines.'

First, in 1617 the apothecaries became independent when King James I granted a charter to form the Society of Apothecaries in recognition of the advances in therapeutics and the development in chemistry. From then on the power of searching the shops of apothecaries within seven miles of London, and examining their drugs, was also vested in their chartered body. The apothecaries had formerly been incorporated with the powerful Guild of Grocers. It was enacted at the same time that no grocer should keep an apothecary's shop, and that no surgeon should sell medicines.

Soon after the apothecaries were formed into a separate society, they took into serious consideration the frauds and artifices practised by the grocers and druggists from whom they obtained their herbs and raw material. In order to remedy this evil they established a central dispensary in 1623, for the purpose of making some of the most important preparations for the use of their own members. This institution was placed under the superintendence of a committee of apothecaries.[6]

All prescriptions had to be filled according to the standards set down by the College of Physicians in their Latin *Pharmacopoeia Londinensis*. The apothecaries now had to set a high standard for their apprentices who could not be accepted without some knowledge of Latin and who had to observe strict rules of conduct. For those who did not live with their masters, there was a dormitory at the Hall over the Master's lodging which was bolted from the outside. These students saw medicines compounded both for physicians and surgeons and, accompanying their masters on their rounds, gained a wider practical experience of therapy than could either a physician or a surgeon.[7] In London, the apothecaries were soon accepted as the general practitioners, particularly since there was a shortage of physicians and, in spite of the tremendous increase in the population of London under the Tudors and early Stuarts, the number of physicians officially accredited by the College of Physicians remained fixed at thirty until 1618 when four royal court physicians were added. The small number could not possibly care for the entire population, and into this void entered apothecaries, doctors with questionable background, 'wisewomen' and quacks. Since the lower classes seldom could afford to pay the fees of the doctors these illegal practioners were largely tolerated.[8]

Although Culpeper was indentured with different masters during the years 1634–1644 he probably was prohibited to sit the examination at the end of his apprenticeship. Obviously his opponents were not only to be found in the Royal College of Physicians but also in the Apothecaries Society.

On the whole the apothecary trade was a disappointment for Culpeper and he did not become a 'free man' (licensee) of the Apothecary Society, or a 'master of the pestle'. He left with the hope of achieving something new, something of his own.

Samuel Leadbetter was three years senior to Culpeper and was freed after being examined on January 9, 1639. Leadbetter also had ideas of his own. When he set up in business Culpeper decided to follow him. Both Culpeper and Leadbetter questioned the conventional practice of the apothecaries of their time, disagreed in matters of composing drugs and designed their own, simpler medicines. Culpeper helped him translate difficult Latin texts and inspired him with new ideas.

An entry in the Apothecaries Court book tells us that Leadbetter had problems with his professional society, it reads: 'Mr. Leadbetter's plaster shall be destroyed. London January 31st, 1642.'

What had happened was this: Leadbetter and Culpeper's business flourished, they sold cheap medicines which probably did not contain all of the expensive ingredients specified in the London Pharmacopoeia, but still did the trick. They also practised medicine helping poor patients. This ignited the envy of the physicians and some apothecaries and led to an official inspection under the supervision of the College of Physicians, who decided that a plaster did not comply with the specifications of the *Pharmacopoeia* and therefore decided it had to be destroyed. That was an unusual decision and is the only one found in the Court Book from 1617 to 1651, therefore we can assume that it was an act of revenge to punish the free-thinking and practising apothecaries.[3]

The early removal in 1642 of royal authority in London left the College of Physicians powerless to enforce its regulation of medical practice and strict censorship practically ceased to exist. The apothecaries, however, probably agreed with the physicians that Culpeper should be stopped in his practice because he was neither examined and approved by the physicians nor the apothecaries. There had, however, been problems before and already in 1634 a battle between the College of Physicians and the Society of Apothecaries came to a head when several apothecaries were accused of practising medicine; specifically mentioned, among others, was Thomas Johnson, the botanist.[9]

The association with Leadbeater continued until 1644 when Culpeper finally decided to set up shop in his own house outside the City walls. This move was preceded by two severe warnings from the Apothecaries Society; on June 3, 1643: 'odered and warned to put away Nicholas Culpeper who so now employed in his shop' and finally, on September 22: 'Mr. Leadbeater is warned not to employ Culpeper in the making or administering of any medicine who promised to obey the same.' Obviously both Culpeper and Leadbeater not only compounded drugs for the physicians but they also in fact 'administered' medicine. It meant that the two received and saw patients. Finally on May 13, 1644: 'Mr. Leadbetter bringing in both parts of the indenture of his apprentice or friend discharged is taken on bond.'

It is quite obvious that both Leadbetter and Culpeper openly engaged in medical practice in the north of London. So, therefore, was it fair to accuse Culpeper of being engaged in illicit medical practice? Was he the naughty quack that his critics say he was?

In order to make a fair judgment we have to assess the role of 17th-century apothecaries. When we speak today about Culpeper as an apothecary we equate this with the profession of a pharmacist preparing medicines only. In most countries, except England, Wales and Ireland, the titles 'apothecary' and 'pharmacist' were virtually interchangeable. The reason for the exception in England being that in the mid-seventeenth century the apothecaries gradually changed from the practice of dispensing to that of practising medicine, and Culpeper was only one of the pioneers in this transition.

Several reasons were responsible for the emancipation of the apothecaries: economic, the scarcity of doctors, and the great plague. Physicians obviously charged much more than the lower educated apothecaries. A university education of twelve years – even though it may not have been very effective – was much more expensive than to be indentured for seven years as an apotheacry apprentice. The number of physicians belonging to the privileged Royal College was limited and there were only few physicians outside the City limits.

In times of crisis, like the great plague of London in 1665, the apothecaries proved to be reliable supporters of the sick when the physicians fled. This finally established their reputation and their role as general practitioners could no longer be questioned. In 1704 the apothecaries in England and Wales finally gained the right to practice medicine, and in 1815 the Apothecaries Act gave them complete control of general practice. The practice of dispensing and compounding medicines passed to the pharmacists or chemists. Eventually the apothecary became the forerunner of the family doctor of later days.

One reason why Culpeper was not more harshly persecuted by the College of Physicians was the 'Quack's Charter' which goes back to 1542. In essence it permitted 'any herb or herbs, ointments, baths, pultess and emplaisters' to be administered for 'a pin and the web in the eye, uncomes of hands, burnings, scaldings, sore mouths, the stone, strangury, saucelim and morphew and such other like disesases'. The only restrictions being that treatment had to be without charge and only externally employed.[10]

5
Encounter with Lilly

The world wishes to be deceived.

Sebastian Brant, 1458–1521

We have good reasons to believe that Culpeper met the most notorious astrologer of his time, William Lilly (1602–1681). Lilly was
Culpeper's senior and had already established a reputation when
he came to London for his apprenticeship. During his formative
years Culpeper was most certainly influenced by him and since
Lilly shared the same puritan political view during this period, it
is very likely that he was his tutor in matters concerning astrology.
In 1651 Culpeper wrote: 'you are all bound to bless God for raising
up that famous man, Mr. William Lilly who has through God's
assistance made the art astrology so plain to you, that you may not
only see your former ignorance, but be in a capacity to do yourselves
good.'[1]

In later years, however, the two were maybe at odds and not on
good speaking terms, since Culpeper is not included in the list of
famous astrologers which Lilly appended to his *Christian Astrology*
of 1659.[2]

William Lilly, of modest origin and upbringing, was born in 1602.
He was an intelligent man and from childhood on obsessed with
dreams and revelations. He had some grammar school knowledge
of Latin and Greek when he came to London to become the personal
servant of a rich merchant, Gilbert Wright. On the death of his master he married his widow, who provided him well, so that he could
spend his time in angling, hearing puritan sermons and learning
astrology from the famed Rhys Evans of Gunpowder Alley.

When Culpeper met him he had already attained the reputation
and fame as an apt astrologer who could cast nativities and predict
future events. He lived on the Strand over against Strand Bridge,

and after the death of his first wife he remarried another rich widow,
Jane, a lady with a sharp tongue.[3]

For a long time Culpeper had wished to see him and one November day in 1635 he decided to pay him a visit. It was a Sunday
afternoon, a bright and cold day, when Culpeper walked down to
the Strand where he had heard that Lilly lived. He inquired at the
nearest inn and upon his question he was immediately given a reply
as to the direction, because Lilly was well known and people seemed
to have a frightful respect for the man. The house was past the
Temple and towards Charing Cross.[4] There he lived in a big corner
house facing south, four stories high with a protruding facade and
many paned windows. On the outside of the third floor was a big
sun-dial.

After knocking the door was opened by a man servant who asked
him about his business. After introducing himself, Culpeper was
shown into the parlour. He looked around and found a room
nicely decorated with guilded leather tapestry above and wooden
panels below. There was a big ornate fireplace with warming
flames, wooden chests and cupboards near the sides and at the
far end a small virginal and a lute on the wall. An elderly lady
appeared, saying that she was the mistress of the house, asked
him again in a shrieky voice for his business and bade him sit
down.

After a while Lilly appeared. He was a man of middle age with
long hair and a severe face. When Culpeper told him that he had
always admired his work, Lilly began to smile and offered to show
him his observatory which was on the top floor. After climbing
three flights of stairs, they came to a big chamber with many high
windows on two sides.

Here a man busied himself writing horoscope charts. Lilly introduced him as his assistant, Mr. Ferdinand Parkhurst. The room was
filled with various instruments for the study of the stars: a long
tube near the window, pointing to the skies, an instrument with
circular rings arranged in a sphere, and two globes. The tables and
the walls were covered by charts of various kinds. Culpeper had
never seen so many implements used solely for the study of the
skies. Only in the attic at Emmanuel College in Cambridge had he
seen a small tube with magnifying glasses which could be used at
night to observe the stars. He stared with surprise and admiration
at all this.

Lilly was only too happy to explain the novelties:

'This,' he said, 'is an astrolabium,' pointing at the glittering arches of circular rings arrranged in a sphere and with scales embossed on the metal.

'And this is a telescope from master Zacharias Jansen of Middleburg in Holland. It is of the latest and best design after the drawings of John Kepler. The two globes you see here on the right represent the earth and the skies. The skye or celestial globe is called an armillary sphere, designed by the great Tycho Brahe, Kepler's teacher. It was brought to England by our late King James I when he visited Brahe at his observatory Uranienborg on the island on Hven in Denmark. King James gave it to his College at Chelsea. When the College was disbanded for religious controversies the many books went to Trinity College and I was lucky to acquire the globe. All these instruments are for the proper study and erudition of astrology, and everything is for the the good of mankind as will be revealed by me.'

'On this chart you can see the planets, which are those heavenly bodies that revolve in orbits around the sun. They are the dependents of the sun, to distinguish them from the thousands of luminous bodies, the fixed stars which stud the sky, and which present to the naked eye no indication of change of place. The planets move sometimes from west to east and sometimes in the opposite direction. It is the study of these movements which are all important for the fate of the earth and its inhabitants.'

Culpeper was deeply impressed and asked:

'I have been reading about starcraft since I was a boy, but nobody, really, told me the art of astrology. How do you use all these instruments and how do you interpret the results?'

'The science and art of astrology to predict terrestrial events by means of the heavenly bodies is simple; look here at the globe and divide the celestial sphere into twelve sectors, or houses of heaven. These houses belong to certain planets which have peculiar powers. This is very similar to the inner surface of a pealed orange. Place the axis of the fruit horizontally in a north and south line, then the divisions of its surface will represent their position on the most common system. If the axis be inclined so as to point either to the pole of the equator or ecliptic, it will show the houses on less common planes. The houses are fixed in position and the planets in their diurnal and orbital movements thus pass from one to another, traversing them all in a day. The power of the houses depends on their position, the one containing the stars about to rise being most powerful and profitable, being the ascendent position. The houses also depend on their subject matter such as life, riches, health, death, friends and enemies etc. Certain houses also belong to certain planets which have particular power.'[2]

'You as an apothecary and physician, you should consult the planetary influence in each patient, to regulate your prescription accordingly. In that case I am persuaded that more immediate relief will in most cases be afforded to the sick and languishing patient. Astrological science should be very useful in guiding your medical enquiries to promote the cure of overt and latent diseases.'

Lilly advanced to the table where he had peculiar square sheets of paper, divided into twelve triangular sectors and one central square. Into these signs were scribbled dates and numbers. Next to it he had many books with tables containing numbers of months, days and hours.

'I will teach you how to make an horoscope or erect a figure of heaven. In the first place you have to draw the figure thus, and to know that those twelve empty spaces are by us called the twelve houses of heaven. That square in the middle is to write the day, year and hour of day. The cusp or very entrance to any house is upon the line where you see the figure placed, upon which line you must place the sign and degree of the zodiac, as you find in this table of houses. In erecting a figure, whether of a question or nativity, you are to consider these three things: first the year, month, day of the week, hour or part of the hour of that day; secondly the true place of the sun; thirdly, what hours and minutes in the table of houses do stand on the left hand against the degree of the sun.'

In addition to the actual date and timing a number of corrections had to be made because in protestant England the Julian calendar had not yet been replaced by the Gregorian which changed the onset of the year.

'Look here,' he said, taking a finished horoscope chart,
'This is my ecliptic scheme demonstrated in the horoscope

chart. The fourth house is cancer. It is the house of the moon, and exaltion of Jupiter. In order to predict an event you determine the state of heaven at the appropriate time and match it with the sign of the zodiac for each person. The signs are: Aries, Taurus, Gemini, Cancer, Leo, Virgo, Libra, Scorpio, Sagittarius, Capricornus, Aquarius and Pisces.'[5]

'That really is not so simple as you say, master Lilly, and it will take some sweat to learn the art of this celestial science, just as it took time and tears to learn Latin from your book, which my grandfather gave me as a child.'

'My dear young man, you are mistaken there, I may be famous in astrology, but not in the Latin tongue. That book was written by a different Lilly, who was Master at St. Paul's School.'[6]

'Medical astrology in essence deals with the questions of sympathy and antipathy of signs and planets to be observed according to their transit through each sign. Some are obnoxious and hateful, others are healthful. Next, consider what disease every planet causes under the signs of the zodiac and what parts of the body the planets generally rule. Masculine planets signify the right side and feminine the left Then may the nature and kind of disease be found out by the houses of heaven and by the nature of the signs as fiery, earthy, airy and watery. As for the length of the disease, it may be found out by the nature of the planets, as follows: Saturn causes long sickness, the Sun and Jupiter short, Mars shorter, but acute, Venus mean, Mercury inconstant, as expected; the moon often gives relapses. Other things concern the type of herbs to be given according to their government and virtues, the time and place to be gathered and many other things.'[2]

'Dear master Lilly, let me ask you a simple question,' said Culpeper, 'how can you reconcile being a good Christian and at the same time an astrologer? If everything is written in the stars and we have access to all future events, what does it matter to try hard to live like a Christian, to do our best, to help man, to correct his faults, to make him change his path?'

'Well, I agree with you, that may be a difficult question, but I will tell you that we earthly creatures can fail in our endeavours and hard work and we all make our mistakes. Look at the sky above us!'

He went to open one of the windows. On this November

afternoon the sun had already set and above them in the dark firmament over on the Thames a few stars were visible.

'See the stars above? Despite all charts and calculations I cannot exactly predict everything. Only think of comets with their tails as swords pointing to a place of joy or destruction. These heavenly bodies all have their meaning and purpose, but their movement in the firmament cannot be predicted. Or think of meteors, those shooting stars that appear as luminous bodies descending to earth. Our earth encounters them in its orbital path as fireballs. Now, with the naked eye you cannot perceive all falling stars, but if you look through the telescope you can make out many meteors and sometimes a comet. You may say like John Donne, who used to live with my neighbour on the Strand.'[7]

> 'Go, and catch a falling star
> Get with child a mandrake root,
> Tell me where all past years are,
> Or who cleft the devil's foot.'

When Culpeper left Lilly they parted as best friends. Culpeper admired Lilly's skills and he tried his best to improve his own knowledge in astrology. Lilly presented him with tables or ephemerides of the years 1636–40 to aid in casting figures and he also gave him some aphorisms for physicians.

'I understand that it may take some time to grasp the subject and therefore I invite you to come back to me as often as you like, not only for science, but also music! Do you play any instrument?'

'Yes, but only the flute and I like to sing.'

'That is fine, you may join us then.'

When Culpeper came home he was somewhat perplexed by the multitude of impressions and he was slightly intimidated and frightened as to how he should manage all these complicated calculations. He looked at the aphorisms for physicians where it said:

From the sign of the sixth, the Lord of that house, planets therein placed, and place of heaven and sign wherein the moon is, require the disease or part afflicted, with relation to the ascendent. – The seventh house represents the physician, the tenth his medicine. If the Lord of the seventh be infortunate, the physician, shall not cure; if the tenth house or Lord thereof, his physician is improper. – The fourth house signifies the end of sickness, and whether it will terminate quickly or endure long: fixed signs prolong, common signs vary the disease, moveable ones show an end one way or other quickly.[2]

The same evening he obtained permission of his master to go to one of his favourite watering holes where he met the friendly old surgeon, Mr. Simon Tresblinck. Culpeper was excited and told him about the adventures of the day and that he had visited the venerated and frightful Mr. Lilly. He described his opulent house and his study with all the fancy instruments for ocular inspection of the skies.

Tresblinck laughted, patted him on the shoulder and said:

'Don't believe in that charlatan and dark imposter. He does not need the shining telescopes and globes because he really does not care about the movement of the stars. His knowledge is from obscure and ancient books and his predictions are always equivocal. I cannot understand how you, an aspiring and gifted young man can believe in the black magic of astrology!'

'From my first youth I have been given to studies, encouraged by my grandfather. I am not satisfied only with the knowledge of Latin and Greek, I want to know the reason for everything and therefore I have taken a singular pleasure in the art of the stars and the secrets of nature.'

'And listen good friend, nobody, not even you can deny that we are under the influence of celestial bodies, particularly the planets like Mercury, Jupiter and Saturn. In everyday life we accept the augurial concepts of people being mercurial, jovial, saturnine. Yes, and you certainly are saturnine, I am mercurial, I am gay and agile and you are more solemn and sober. And don't we say and accept the notion that a mad man is under the influence of the moon or lunatic?'

'Yes, that may be, but it is only everyday talk and proves nothing. In his book, *Anatomy of Melancholy*, Robert Burton tells us that there are physicians that do not believe more in the celestial signs as they do in the signs of an innkeeper's

post or tradesman's shop but others, like Paracelsus is of
the opinion that a physician without the knowledge of stars
can neither understand the cause or cure of any disease. I
agree with Burton, I am convinced that: "They do incline
but not compell and that a wise man may resist them: '*sapiens
dominatur astris*". They rule us, but God rules them. The heaven
is God's instrument, a great book, whose letters are the stars,
wherein are written many strange things for such as can read.
Or an excellent harp, made by an eminent workman, on which
he that can play, will make most admirable musik.'[8]

'Don't you believe in the holy Bible, and the magi who came
to the birth of Christ? These were astrologers and physicians!
Matthew tells us three wise men came from Babylon to Jeru-
salem, led by a star guiding them safely to Christ's place
of birth in Bethlehem. There they offered gold, frankincense
and myrrh. These gifts were nothing but precious medicines
to preserve the health of the holy child.'

'In our calendar the three days after New Year's Day bear the
names of the magi or kings, Kaspar, Melchior and Balthasar,
and their memory is preserved in the feast of the three holy
kings – the Epiphany.'

'I can see that it is hard to convince you about the vanity of
astrology. You will have to find out the truth for yourself by
experience and maybe painful lessons.'

Lilly was an opportunist and skilful political manipulator who
always floated on the waves of the prevailing political currents,
a successful propagandist for the Parliamentarians and prophet of
their victories, and later pretended to be a loyal follower of the
King. His predictions were vague, but he was shrewd enough to
occasionally stumble on something that was plausible. He was a
forcaster of evil events like eclipses, the Great Fire of London in 1665
and the Great Plague of 1666. He ended his career by being licensed
in 1670 to practice medicine by the Archbishop of Canterbury and
died in 1681 at the age of 79.

6

Alice Field

So wise so young, they say, do never live long.
William Shakespeare, 1564–1616

Many times Arthur Dee, Ferdinand Parkurst and Nicholas Culpeper met at Lilly's house – all men with a common interest: the stars and musik. One day they were sitting at the table in the study, looking at the notebook of John Dowland. Lilly was playing the lute and they sung quartetto:

> 'Awake sweet love thou art returned,
> my hart which long in absence mournd
> lives now in perfect joy.'

Lilly said to Culpeper: 'You seem so happy today like no day before. What happened, are the planets favourable to you?'

'My heart rejoices and I can sing again with mirth, I have found a new love. Before I could not sing with joy the many love songs we had.'[1]

What happened was that he had met the charming Alice Field whom he married in 1640:

He was courted by his friends to alter the condition of his single life, he would admit to no such proffers, till like a skilful astrologer he had fixed his eyes upon the firmament, where Venus, the star of his own affections governed, surrendering all the powers and faculties of his soul to the vertues and beauty of Miss Alice Field.[2]

The chosen one was a fifteen-year-old lass, pretty and probably impressed by the temperamental Culpeper with his piercing dark eyes. Culpeper met his future bride through his medical practice.

He was called to the house of Charles Field, a grain merchant near
Aldersgate. Mr. Field was troubled with gouty arthritis and suffered
intense pain in the great toe and ankle. He had tried everything and
spent large sums of money for consultations. Alice had been running
with urine specimens to different physicians and without even
seeing the patient they prescribed expensive nostrums and made
additional house calls to administer *venesectio* (bleeding). When
nothing helped Field decided to call Culpeper, whose reputation
as a marvellous healer was well known. When Culpeper came to
Field's house he was received by Alice who ushered him to the
living quarters. Culpeper did his best and prescribed a poultice
of barley which 'easeth the hot pains of the gout' and roots of
cinquefoil boiled in wine, because 'applied to the joints full of
ache and pains doth cure them'. After these therapeutic attempts
the swelling eased and Charles Field decided he wanted to take
the waters at the newly established spa of Tunbridge Wells. Alice
accompanied him and he invited Culpeper to join them. The trip to
Tunbridge Wells took Culpeper away from the pressures of work
and for the first time in years he could relax. It gave him a chance
to realise that life had more to offer than work and worries. He felt
relieved and happy and an important reason was Alice. Was it love
at first sight? Was she chosen because of a favourable horoscope?
Was it an arranged match?

'A gentlewoman of good extraction, so also besides her richer
qualities, her admirable discretion and excellent breeding, she
brought him considerable fortune.' What shall we think of this?
If it were not a love match, was he impressed by her dowry,
since it is mentioned by Ryves both with regards to his first young
love Judith and now with Alice.[2] In the seventeenth century the
selection of a partner was a very serious decision. Social class,
political views, family recognition etc. had to be considered and
economic factors certainly played a great role. There is ample
evidence for this. In Dorothy Osborne's (1627–1695) letters we are
informed that:

> My cousin Franklin left a gentleman, whom she had much
> more kindness for than ever she had for Mr. Franklin, because
> his estate was less and suffered herself to be persuaded that
> twenty-three hundred pound a year was better than twelve,
> though with a person she loved; and has recovered it so well,
> that you see her confess there is nothing in her condition she

desires to alter at the charge of a wish. She's happier by much than I shall ever be.[3]

Anything less or more than an arranged marriage was frowned upon. How should young people recognise a suitable partner? Society gladly accepted the alliance of forty-five year old Francis Bacon (1561–1626) when he married the fourteen-year-old rich heiress Alice Barnham. But we know that the poet John Donne (1572–1631) wrecked his career when he ran away with the sixteen-year-old daughter of his employer, Sir Thomas Egerton, 'dressed charmingly as a page' – the standard costume of young women embarking on such adventures.[4]

The recipe for a happy marriage was, according to the seventeenth-century proverb, 'Marry first and love will come after.'[5]

It was important that the match was carefully prepared and approved by everybody concerned. Culpeper had already learned this by painful experience when he lost his first love.

The marriage with Alice Field must have been a happy one, at least for Culpeper, since we are informed that:

> Mrs Culpeper while she continnued in that blessed state of matrimony fourteen years with him she so wisely demeand herself, as never to entrench on his prerogative, not in the least to disturb his studies; she only sought to maintain her own propriety in domestic feminine affairs; so that she was all his time a wife at her own disposing, enfranchised, free-born from her wedding day.[2]

In 1640 when Nicholas married Alice Field he moved north 'without Bishopsgate' (outside the City Wall) not far from Threadneedle Street to Spitalfields. He had obtained a large dowry and could afford to build his own house near Spitalsquare. From this square we enter Red and White Lion Streets. On Red Lion Street 'next to the Red Lion'. (See plate of his house). The house had rooms downstairs for receiving patients and where medicines could be compounded, and upstairs bedrooms and a study. In the small house next door his assistant (Mr. William Ryves) and servants probably lived upstairs. He may also have added a garden for medicinal herbs.

Bishopsgate in the east of London was close to Leaden Hall with the nearby Herb Market, and not far from the wharfs. The area around Bishopsgate had names which have associations with pharmacy, such as Wormwood Street, Camomille Street and Lime Street. This sounds very idyllic indeed but anyone approaching Bishopsgate must have been frightened by a horrid view: the portal was adorned with poles mounted on the corner turrets which carried joints of flesh that were once quarters and limbs of convicted 'traitors' whose heads had been displayed on the south entrance of London Bridge. After leaving Bishopsgate one came to a sparsely populated rural area, a district on the fringe of the strict jurisdiction of the City which therefore enjoyed certain liberties and invited the establishment of the first permanent London scenes as 'The Theatre' and 'Curtain' and various dubious amenities like pleasure grounds such as 'Fisher's Folly' with bowling alleys and Beargardens.[6]

The area northeast of Bishopsgate was called Moorfields. As the name indicates, this was a wet, fenny place, for a long time unsuitable for large buildings but used as 'tenter grounds' given over to laundresses who hanged their linen sheets like tents to dry and bleach in the open. The fields were full of wild flowers and herbs. Hampstead Heath in the northwest was frequently mentioned in herbals by Gerard, Johnson and Culpeper. The stretch of pasture immediately north of the Moorfields and east of Finsbury Court was called Mallow Field, presumably taking its name from the pale mallow-flowers praised by Culpeper.

On Thursdays the song of laundresses and birds was interrupted by thunder and explosions which came from the nearby Old Artillery Yard, the training grounds for the gunners from the nearby Tower who, in testing their newest equipment, made the houses shudder with explosions.[6] This was in sharp contrast to the idyllic and peaceful rural picture of the Moorfields and Spitalfields.

When the Culpepers came to Spitalfields this was still a scarcely populated area in the north-east of London. The name came from a priory and house of charity, 'St Mary Spittel without Bishopsgate' that existed there, until in 1534 Henry VIII dissolved the institution, pulled down the buildings and gave the ground to one Stephen Vaugn. The Spital itself was located at the northern side of Spital Square, a plot of land with a pulpit, that once belonged to the spital, and was devoted to open air preaching.

The tradition of preaching at Spital Square persisted even after the dissolution of the priory, and the pulpit was used for the celebrated Spital-sermons, regularly preached at Easter time and attended not only by locals, but also by most of the important people in the City. In 1617 the archbishop of Canterbury and the great Lord Bacon came to hear the gospel preached. Near the south side of the pulpit was a house for the accomodation of the Lord Mayor, the Aldermen, their ladies and persons of distinction from the court end of the town. The pulpit was finally destroyed in the Civil War.

At other times fairs were held in Spital Square and according to a broadside, both Lilly and Culpeper had exhibits at them. Fairs were quite popular and attracted huge crowds of people, who at the same time probably also frequented Culpeper's nearby apothecary shop.

Spitalfields was a rapidly expanding area with a mostly poor population which later received Dutch and French immigrants, living in simple houses. Many of these brought with them the art of silk spinning and weaving. Nothing is left of these old places in Spitalfields and today part of the area is occupied by Liverpool Street Station. The site of Culpeper's house is near Fournier Street, next to Christ Church.

At about the same time he married, his grandfather, the reverend William Attersoll, died and was buried on May 30, 1640. His grandson had been a disappointment to him: 'Attersol had formerly used his best arguments, though to no purpose to persuade him to embrace the ministerial function, with an intention as it was supposed after his decease to have settled his estate on him; which he since would not hearken too, he divided four hundred pounds a year amongst the rest of his grandchildren and left him but a legacy of forty shillings, which was paid him by two executors at Nathaniel Brook his shop at the Angell in Cornhill. This small summe he received with a smile, and said, he had courted two mistresses that had cost him very dear, but that it was not the wealth of kingdoms should buy them from him.'[2]

Nathaniel Brook was a printer and bookseller with whom Attersoll must have had business. The same Brook later published some of Culpeper's books.

His experience in the East End of London with its poor population made Culpeper realise that treatment had to be affordable and cheap. Because of this and his puritan views he came to embrace wholeheartedly the dogma of 'English herbs for English bodies', a view that had been introduced by the Elizabethan physician Timothy Bright[7] and was shared by Thomas Johnson, the editor of the second edition of Gerard's *Herbal*. He expressed the opinion that: 'I verily believe that the divine Providence had a care in bestowing Plants in each part of the Earth, fitting and convenient to the forknown necessities of the future inhabitants; and if we thoroughly knew the vertues of these, we needed no Indian or American Drugges.'8

Culpeper practised mainly among the poor and needy and prescribed cheap and 'healthy' medicines made of flowers and plants that grew nearby. Culpeper never denied treating anybody rich or poor and often had 40 patients a day. He took his time listening to his patients:

> Many a times I find my patients disturbed by trouble of conscience and sorrow and I have to act the divine before I can be a physician. In fact our greatest skils lies in the infusion of hopes, to induce confidence and peace of mind.

At the beginning of the seventeenth century regulations about medical education and practice were particularly strict in London. In 1595 it had been decreed that: 'No surgeon, no man, though never so learned a physician or doctor, might practise in London, or within seven miles, without the licence of the College of Physicians.'

In the provinces it was much easier. Professional guilds could include physicians, apothecaries and surgeons and therefore must be regarded as the early nurseries of general practice.[7]

Culpeper certainly knew about this regulation and, although outside the city walls, he lived within the seven-mile city limit. As we have seen already during his apprenticeship he disregarded the rule and always was full of contempt for his learned colleagues. More and more he developed a critical view about the physicians and their obscure craft.

The standard of seventeenth-century therapeutics was medieval and the established physicians could easily be criticised:

> They are bloodsuckers, true vampires, have learned little since Hippocrates; use bloodletting for ailments above the midriff and purging for those below. They evacuate and revulse their patients until they faint. Black hellebor, this poisonous stuff, is a favourite laxative. It is surprising that they are so pupular and that some patients recover. My own poor patients would not endure this taxing and costly treatment. The victims of physicians only survive since they are from the rich and robust stock, the plethoric red skinned residents of Cheapside, Westminster and St James.

Happily married and settled in Spitalfields he finally separated from Samuel Leadbetter (who had developed sympathies for the Royal College of Physicians) and developed his own profile. He soon developed a reputation as a radical healer and attracted pupils. One of them was William Ryves.

In order to make progress radical change was necessary and Culpeper now embarked on this road. An implicit faith in the opinion of the tradition of teaching, an attachment to systems and established forms, and a dread of reflexions, have always followed those who practise medicine as a trade. Few improvements were to be expected from a man who might ruin his reputation, very existence and family by even the smallest deviation from the established rule. Therefore it is fair to realise that in the seventeenth century few valuable discoveries in medicine were made by accepted physicians. They were in general either the result of chance or neccessity and usually opposed by contemporary authorities.

> These judges of physick in their splendor assume a mask of gravity and importance to hide their ignorance. But in our times of illumination and freedom from popery and doctrine, laity have asserted their rights to inquiry into subjects of religion and science. Why should not everybody have these same rights to inquire into medicine, a subject that seriously affects everybody's life?[9]

He also was in favour of careful examination. The diagnostic procedures were strange and among the established physicians one of the most important tests was uroscopy or water casting. This was done by inspecting a urine flask or urinal which sometimes was brought to the physician so that he could make his diagnosis *par distance*, without having to see the patient eye-to-eye. The urine was always contained in a characteristic flask, and this was carried in an osier basket with lid and handle, looking very much like a champagne bucket. The urinal became the emblem of medical practice, and was even in some places used as a sign-board.[10]

Culpeper's view about uroscopy was: 'drawn from the urine is as brittle as the urinal' and proper investigation 'is a better way to find the disease than viewing the piss, though a man should view as much as the Thames will hold.'[11]

To his amanuensis Ryves he complained:

'I tell you about a patient treated by a physician. I was called as a last resort to his deathbed. He had been taken ill with a severe shaking ague. Bleeding was the only treatment he received, apart from antimony powder, which made him worse. They drew pint after pint until he lost his consciousness. I came too late, could help nothing, only comfort his wife. They think that bleeding will relieve all dycrasias and that this can restore the disturbed balance of most anything. This they call derivation. Galen himself mentions that if a patient is bleeding to death from one part of the body, open a vein in another, and the bleeding from the first will stop.'

Ryves replied:

'Many think of you as a coward, who does not dare or have the skill to use the lancet. They say you are so thin and feeble that you swoon and faint as soon as you see blood'.

'First of all I do not believe in bleeding and secondly this is something for butchers and barbers.'

The judgment ot the physicians of the Royal College about Culpeper certainly was not favourable either: 'He pretends to be a doctor, just because he can warble some Latin and Greek, but in reality he does not even have a Pots Hall (apothecary) degree.'

Culpeper had an inquisitive mind and was never satisfied with his achievements. He was driven with a burning desire for achievement. When he was not seeing patients he wrote medical tracts.

At that time Culpeper already had taken up the habit of smoking and he was often chastised by his friends for using this poison. 'The destructive tobacco Mr. Culpeper too excessively took. Tobacco was the greatest enemy he had to his health, but he was too much accustomed to it, to leave it.'[2]

It is surprising that Culpeper was an avid smoker because it neither fits with his medical principle which was against using foreign herbs nor with his puritan views he had adopted after he began a new life after Judith's tragic death. The reason was simply that he was irrevocably addicted to the vice. Moreover, Culpeper was himself at the source of cheap tobacco since sellling was chiefly taken over by the apothecaries whose shops became meeting places or 'ordinaries' of smokers. Druggists and apothecaries were also well stocked with other smoking paraphenelia such as Winchester clay pipes, maple blocks for cutting tobacco and juniper wood for charcoal fires. The pipes were lit with a tinder stick or pieces of glowing charcoal which were held with a silver tong to the smoker's pipe.

Tobacco was introduced to Britain in 1586 by Sir Walter Raleigh and it very soon became very popular so that it was placed under duty already in Elizabeth's reign at 2 d per pound. The duty was raised to 6 s 10 d by James I. In 1620 the growing of tobacco in England was officially prohibited and in 1624 there was a further proclamation confirming that no tobacco was to be grown in the realm but that it could be imported from Virginia, though at high import duties.

Tobacco became an important part of every dispensatory including the *Pharmacopoeia Londinensis*. It was used for a variety of ailments such as migraine, asthma and flegm of the lungs and also against parasites. Culpeper particularly praises it for its ability to kill worms, ' . . . this I know by experience, even when all other medicines have failed'.[12]

Smoking was an issue of great controversy, and four treatises had appeared to condemm the habit.[cf. 13,14] King James himself had participated in the polemics when he published: *A counterblast to tobacco*. His majesty had proclaimed: 'Smoking tobacco is like hell in the very substance of it, for it is a stinking loathsome thing; and so is hell.' King James' diatribe was published anonymously in 1604, and its authorship was only disclosed twelve years later. James felt a sense of moral responsibility and he believed that the words that flowed from his exalted pen would be taken seriously:

> Medicine has the vertue that it never leaveth a man in the state wherein it findeth him, it makes a sick man whole, but a whole man sick. And as medicine helpeth nature being taken at times of necessitie, so being ever and continually used, it doth but weaken, wearie and weare nature. It was first found out by some of the barbarous Indians, to be a preservative, or antidot against the Pockes, a filthy disease, whereunto these barbarous people are (as all men know) very much subject, what through the uncleanly and adust constitution of their bodies, and what through intemperate heate of their climate so that as from them was was first

brought into Christendome, that most detastable disease, so from them likewise was first brought this use of tobacco, as a stinking and unsavorie antidot, for so corrupted and execrable a maladie, the stinking suffumigation, whereof they yet use against that disease, making so one canker or vemine to eate out another.

One tract was called: *Worke for Chimny-Sweepers*. Two appeared in 1616, one by John Deacon: *Tobacco tortured*, in the form of a dialogue between a proponent, Capnistus, and the wise Hydrophorus who in the strongest words condemmed the use of tobacco. Raphael Thorius heroically defended the use of tobacco. He wrote the *Hymos Tabaci* in praise of tobacco at a time when the plant was being castigated by James I and his followers. This poem was circulated among 'cultured English society'.

One anonymous physician dared to present what he called: *A defence of Tobacco*[15] and Edmund Gardiner in 1611 published a lengthy treatise about the medicinal virtues of the tobacco plant. He talked about 'smokie medicine' but at the same time hinted at the addicting properties when he gave the fitting description:

> How great the force and power of this cruel tyrant custome is, that creepeth in little by little, insinuating himself slily into our natures, so at length he will be malepart, as to vindicate the whole rule and government of our bodies, prescribing and limiting new law, even such itself pleaseth.

It is significant to note that Gardiner (1611) in his enthusiastic description of the medicinal virtues of tobacco mixed recent experience of this plant from the New World with the quotations of classical authors. In the beginning of his book he includes a list of two separate pages with 74 names of 'authors and learned men whose authorities are cited in this present Worke'. In order to make his arguments convincing he reverently quotes Homeros, Albertus Magnus, Galen, Hippocrates, Paracelsus, although these men had absolutely nothing to do with Nicotiana or Tobacco.[16]

Culpeper may have realised the danger of smoking and it should have been contrary to his principles of using a foreign herb, but this did not stop him, probably both due to addiction and because he was a strong individualist who always went his own way; moreover, he was anti-royal, particularly against the bigot James I and the self-centered Charles I. In fact, it probably made him feel good to blow out tobacco fumes when it was known that the habit was forbidden by kings, popes and sultans.

One of the reasons why tobacco as a medicinal plant in England became such an immediate success was the English translation of the book by the Spaniard from Seville, Nicolas Monardes, *Joyfull Newes out of the New found World*. It had become immensely popular with physicians and apothecaries. The text praised the virtues of the new imported medicines.[17]

William Ryves, his collaborator and amanuensis who had criticised his master for smoking tobacco and who certainly knew about Monardes and the new drugs from the West Indies said: 'Why do you use tobacco rather than the new balsamo and guaiac-oil?' To this his master replied:

'William, read the book carefully and you will find the proper use for Monardes drugs. Look here what it says':

'In the island of Sancto Domingo was an Indian who gave knowledge thereof to his master, in this manner. A Spaniard that did suffer great paines of the Poxe, which he had by the company of an Indian women, but his servant being one of the physicians of that country, gave unto him the water of guaiacan, wherewith not only were his grievous paines taken away that he did suffer: but healed very well of the evill with which many other Sparniards that were infected with the same evill were healed. The knowledge of this was communicated immediately, with them that came from thence and it was divulged throughout all Spaine, and from there through all the world. With most certainty, it healeth and cureth the said disease, without turning to fall again, except the sick man do return to tumble in the same bosome, where he took the first. – Our Lord GOD would from whence the evill of the Poxe came, from thence send the remedy for them. For the Pox came into these partes from Indias, and first of all from Sancto Domingo.'[17]

'This man, Monardes is a sensible and learned physician and even though he adheres to popish teachings he understands the laws of God's providence to provide medicine at the right time and the right place.'

'So, William, if I see a patient with Indian Poxe I will send for Indian medicine, like guaiac-oil.'

'But master, don't you approve of the many medicinal virtues of the tobacco plant mentioned in this very same excellent book?'

'No, only for certain ailments such as killing of lice, as advocated by Monardes. We have excellent simples for other diseases in England. – English herbs for English people.'

7

Civil War & Fights

A few honest men are better than numbers.

Oliver Cromwell, 1599–1658

O horse, O horse, O bully Graham
and pray do get thee far from me with speed,
and get thee out o' this country quite,
that no one may know who has done the deed.

17th-century broadsheet.

The Puritan revolution was also the age of John Milton, its foremost poet and prophet. This was the time of the awakening of the human mind to a full consciousness of its rights to freedom of thought and freedom of imagination. The commotions of the Civil War were, as he perceived, the pains and agonies which accompanied the birth of a new society, although not quite of the type he desired and had hoped for. Milton's writings, as expressed in his pamphlets, are the voice of liberty, religious, private and political, which would reconcile the conflicting force. His dictum: 'Liberty . . . is the nurse of all great wits!' certainly was an ideal to which Culpeper also subscribed. Milton's age, however, became one of disintegration, when the weakening of accepted principles and the rise of new modes of thought resulted in an intellectual as well as social upheaval.[1]

Culpeper can clearly be looked upon as part of this spiritual process of liberation, and it is therefore not surprising that he participated in the battlefield on the Parliamentarian side.

Politically, the Civil War was the result of a long conflict between the people's Parliament and an estranged monarch and his religious ambitions. The commotions of the Civil War were felt all over Britain. To Puritan protestants and the Calvinist Scots, both the monarch and his archbishop, Laud, were guilty of popish innovations which could be a prelude to a return to Rome. There was also the question of taxation: ship money horrified a great part of the English gentry. Londoners were discontent with the King, merchants saw their trade restricted and citizens were worried by rising prices. The reason was that Charles I granted monopolies to his favourites and courtiers, thereby increasing his influence and receiving extra revenues. When, in 1642, a confrontation became inevitable, King Charles left London. He moved from Hampton Court to York to find support for his cause. Parliament had taken over government in London and under their leader, the Earl of Essex, mobilised the people against monarchy.

Meanwhile the King also had enlisted an army in the north and raised his standard at Nottingham where he was met by his German nephews Prince Rupert, the 'mad cavalier', and his brother Maurice.

Essex left London in September and joined forces with a troop of horse led by captain Oliver Cromwell from Cambridge. The first battle in the Civil War between Parliament and King Charles I which eventually produced the Commonwealth and the Cromwellian Protectorate was that of Edgehill in 1642.[2-5]

The call for volunteers met Culpeper in London and he immediately replied by going to the recruitment centre near the Royal Exchange at Cornhill. There he offered his service to take part in the battle. When he was asked about his profession he explained that he was an apothecary and practitioner. The recruitment officer said: 'We do not need you at the battle front but you can come along as a field surgeon, since most of the barbers and physicians are royalist asses and we have use for someone to look after our wounded.'[6]

During the Civil War physicians, with the exception of a small number known by name, were not regularly appointed to the fighting services, but towards the middle of the seventeenth century apothecaries were recruited.

So it was decided, and Culpeper prepared himself for the journey north with the convoy of troops. He had always wanted to be a real physician, approved by the Royal College of Physicians, but he had never dreamt of becoming a surgeon. He was not much inclined towards bloody butchery and to him it was a barbarous but necessary trade. He had never had any clashes with members of that profession; in fact, he even used to send some patients to Mr. Tersman, the barber in Spitalfields, for stonecutting and setting of broken bones. In order to prepare himself he borrowed the book *Opera Chirurgica* by the famous French military surgeon, Ambroise Paré. Nicholas with his usual determination studied the Latin text with great fervour. He also assembled some simple instruments and bandages in a medicine box.

When Culpeper started his march north to receive orders from his superior, he passed through Hatfield, St Albans, Dunstable, and Northampton up to Edgehill. On his way he did not miss the opportunity to look for medicinal herbs which he collected and described in a diary. He had the opportunity to stay at Gorhambury near St Albans, the residence of the much admired Francis Bacon who died there in pursuit of natural science. (In March of 1626 Bacon caught a cold while stuffing a fowl with snow near Highgate, in order to observe the effect of cold on the preservation of flesh.)[6]

The battle at Edgehill took place the next month and William Harvey was attached to the King's family as attendant physician, so that we had the royalist Harvey on one side and the Puritan-Parliamentarian Culpeper on the other side of the front.[6]

The battle ended without a definite victor. The King and his soldiers marched to Oxford and then towards London where he took Reading and proceeded to Turnham Green, just upriver from Putney. But here he was finally stopped by a big army, newly recruited in London. Thereupon the King retreated to Oxford for the winter and Culpeper returned to London. Back at home in Spitalfields Alice cried and lamented that her husband had joined the war but Culpeper said. 'Cursed be every man that goes not out, cursed be every wife that consents not to her husband going out to these wars.'

Negotiations for peace were unsuccessful and in February of 1643 Parliament ordered fortifications of London with ditches and ramparts that surrounded the whole city.

In April, Essex, general of the Parliamentary army, moved forward to Reading which he captured. Culpeper this time felt that his duties were at the front itself. Everything had to be done to stop the King from capturing London.

Culpeper, from his previous engagement, had at least got an idea of what war was all about. He received a commission to be captain of a troop of foot. He raised a company of sixty volunteers, all young men from London. At Reading a spent bullet wounded him in the left shoulder so that he had to be brought back to London in a carriage.[6]

When Culpeper first arrived in London to serve as an apprentice to an apothecary, Nicholas had a letter of recommendation to Lord John Compton of Islingon from his uncle, William Culpeper of Wakehurst. Compton was a distant relative to the Culpepers of Wakehurst and it was thought proper and commendable that young Nicholas might have the assistance and company of this important man, whose estate was not far from Spitalfields. Culpeper was invited several times to the generous household north of London, not far from the deep forests of Middlesex. To begin with these visits were a pleasant distraction and opportunity for Nicholas to mix with society and to taste the good life in a country mansion. The Comptons, however, were strict royalists and at the beginning of the Civil War their relationship became polarised and hostile.

Open conflict started when Culpeper attacked established physicians and royalists. One day in 1646, John Compton, on his way to town, came rumbling in at Spitalfields, probably not sober, and started shouting abuse not only at him but also at Alice, calling her a whore. Culpeper became furious and responded with the same abusive language and a request of an apology else he demanded satisfaction. This was not forthcoming, and both being proud gentlemen there was no other solution than a duel. This was hastily and discreetly arranged to take place the next weekend at Finsbury Fields with John Smith as Culpeper's second. Pistols were chosen as weapons, since Culpeper, incapacitated by his war injuries, was unable to use the sabre.

Early at daybreak both parties dismounted at the far end of the field, away from habitation. Two fateful shots were fired. Culpeper was left unhurt but Compton fell to the ground, wounded in the neck. There was lot of blood gushing from the wound and the assailed fainted. Culpeper dressed the wound, left his friend with the other party, and disappeared in the rainy morning.

When he came home he locked himself up in his study, not admitting anybody. Patients assembled as usual outside the dispensary but waited in vain. In the afternoon Smith came with the news: Compton was severely wounded and his family wanted revenge.

In 1613 private duelling was prohibited by King James I in his 'Proclamation against private Challenges and Combats'. During Queen Elizabeth's reign duelling had reached frightening proportions and young gallants had given up the old-fashioned sword in favour of the newer, more stylish and deadlier rapier. Therefore it had become common practice for duels to be fought abroad. Francis Bacon, the scientist, and at the time solicitor general, delivered to the Star Chamber his 'Charge against duels', requesting to introduce a law prohibiting men to go beyond the sea for the purpose of fighting a duel. Such a law could, however, not be enforced and many young men went to nearby Calais in pursuit of their foolish plans. Duelling being declared a crime, the outcome meant that Culpeper could face imprisonment and even the death penalty.

After the fateful duel at Finsbury Fields with John Compton, Culpeper decided to leave the country quickly in order to evade imprisonment. He told Alice and Smith that he would go to Paris, and asked to be informed about the fate of Compton by messages to be delivered to the English embassy. This was an escape from responsibility, but he also thought that it might give him a chance to realise his wish to visit Riolan, the famous French physician and the astronomer Pierre Gassendi at the College Royal in Paris.[7]

He quickly made the necessary arrangements and informed Alice about his route, and where he intended to stay, in order to receive information about the state of health of his opponent. To avoid problems with free passage and nosy questions from habour guards, he decided to go to Weymouth, and from there to one of the English Channel Islands. In Weymouth Culpeper went aboard a frigate bound for St Peter Port on Guernsey. The ship belonged to the Parliamentary fleet, so there was no danger in crossing to Guernsey which was in Parliamentary hands. After some days waiting he was taken by a Dunkirk privateer to St Malo. On their way they were boarded by a ship from Jersey which was still in Royal hands and where the Prince of Wales stayed before he took refuge in France. The soldiers searched the vessel and when the chief officer looked at Culpeper's papers he saluted and let him go, because he realised that he was a relative of the famous Sir John Culpeper, chancellor of the Exchequer to the King (see Culpeper's pedigree in Figure 1), and presently also in Jersey.[8]

We only know that Culpeper stayed in France for three months and then he probably returned when news reached him about the recovery of his opponent. Did he meet Jean Riolan, the brilliant Parisian anatomist, and Pierre Gassendi, the astronomer? In Culpeper's writings we do not hear anything about Gassendi, and although he criticised Aristotle, he was probably too much of a cool scientific astronomer to attract Culpeper's curiosity. Culpeper, however, later translated one of Riolan's books.

In January 1649 King Charles I was tried for his life and publicly beheaded at Whitehall. His son, the Prince of Wales and now Charles II, returned to England and assumed command of the Royal forces. He was, however, soon defeated and again fled to France.

There were many casualties on both sides of the conflict. It is a tragic irony that King Charles I was legally killed by the highest political authority, Parliament, and that his son Charles II, later after the Restoration, was killed by the highest medical authorities of the time, his court physicians. At least it can be concluded that his death was hastened by bleeding, vomiting, purging and the administrations of cordials containing 'extract of human scull and bezoar stone'. Dr Scarburgh, one of the dozen physicians called to treat the King relates: 'Alas after an ill fated night his serene majesty's strength seemed exhausted to such a degree that the whole assembly of physicians lost all hope and became despondent: still so as not to appear to fail in doing their duty in any detail, they brought into play the most active cordial.' And as a grand conclusion to this pharmaceutical debauch a mixture of Raleigh's antidote, pearl julep, and ammonia, was forced down the throat of the dying king.[9]

Two and a half centuries later therapy was not much different and it is significant to note the fate of the dying Lord Byron in his Greek military campaign, when taken ill by a fever and subjected by his doctors to bleeding and antimony powder. It is probably quite true what he laconically said about people of his class who could afford physicians: 'The lancet has killed more people than the lance'.[10]

One day the same year, Culpeper's daughter, Mary, was feverish, had a swelling on her neck, and no appetite. Culpeper immediately realised that she had developed scrofula or 'King's Evil'.[11] By old English tradition this disease was best cured by the 'Royal Touch'. That meant that the afflicted person after being investigated by the King's surgeon, was brought to his majesty and after a religious ceremony the monarch touched the neck and thereafter placed a coin, an Angel, worth about 10 shillings, on a white ribbon around the neck of the sufferer.[12]

Since there was no longer a king in England who could minister to their child it is therefore not surprising that mother Alice and grandmother Mary became very worried. They opened their heart to Nicholas and asked for his help. He some years later reported in his *English Physitian*:

> What vulgarly is called King's Evil really are swellings or kernels on the neck near the ears which may be broken and running. There are many good remedies for this affliction. I have myself with great success used an ointment made of pilewort to cure my own daughter. It broke the sore! drew out a quarter of a pint of corruption, and cured without any scar at all in a week's time.[11]

Obviously he did not miss the King and his ministrations for this disease.

The tradition of the 'Royal Touch' was introduced by the Anglo-Saxon king Edward the Confessor in the 11th century and was deeply rooted in the minds of English people ever since. The tradition survived the Reformation and was practised by Henry the VIII and Queen Elizabeth I. When James I came from Scotland to take up his English throne, he was anxious to discontinue the practice of touching, expressing disbelief of the transmission of the power from the Confessor. In a letter it was said that 'When some of these patients were presented to him in his ante-chamber, he first had a prayer offered by a Calvinist minister, and then remarked that he was puzzled as to how to act. He did not see how the patient could be cured without a miracle, and nowadays miracles had ceased and no longer happened; so he was afraid of committing a superstitious act. From another point of view, however, inasmuch as it was an ancient usage and for the good of his subjects, he resolved to give it a trial, but only by way of prayer, in which he begged all present to join him, and then he touched the sick folk.'

Under Charles I's rule the practice of the Royal Touch grew in frequency and popularity partly because of his marriage to the French princess Henrietta Maria, who had long been accustomed to the ceremony from the French court, and since he did not want to forgo any of the prerogatives of sovereignity. New touch-pieces were issued under his reign and numerous proclamations made to invite citizens for his healing sessions. These proclamations, besides being publicly exposed in every market town, were to be read in every church twice a year and churchwardens of each parish were instructed to see that the proclamation was permanently displayed in the church. During Culpeper's time the belief in the Royal healing not only for scrofula but also for other afflictions reached hysterical proportions. Wherever King Charles dwelt in the Kingdom, either as monarch or prisoner, people followed him and sought his healing power. Many cures were said to have been brought about by handkerchiefs and cloths dipped in the blood of the King at his execution.

Under the Protectorate of Oliver Cromwell the practice of the Royal Touch ceased to exist but an Irishman, Valentine Greatrakes, became obsessed with the idea that he was given the royal and divine power to heal by stroking. For some time he practised faith healing not only for the 'King's Evil' but also for many other maladies.[12]

8

Pandora's Box, 1649

Go, take physic, dote upon
Some big-named composition,
The oraculous doctors' mystic bills-
Certain hard words made into pills;
And what at last shalt thou gain by these?
Only costlier disease.

Richard Crashaw, 1613–1649

In 1648 at Christmas time Anthony and Elisabeth Parris came to visit their nephew Nicholas and his wife Alice. They had travelled all the way up from Isfield, Sussex, to London.[1]

Under the Puritan Commonwealth Christmas and May Day celebrations had been abandoned and stage plays, church ales and gambling were forbidden by law. Fiddlers and minstrels found in taverns were declared vagabonds and treated as such.[2] But in most houses the Christmas traditions with plenty of food and drink were still maintained and merry England was not destroyed in the house of the Culpepers in Spitalfields. Alice busied herself at Christmas-time. She made decorations with bay, holly, ivy and mistletoe, baked and roasted. Alice called upstairs:

'Please Nicholas, come down and enjoy the feast'.

He finally made a move and walked down to the illuminated room which was filled by the nice smells of herbs, cakes and other sweetmeats. He sat down by the fire.

Anthony said:

'What occupies you so intensely day and night in your study?'

'I am writing for the press a translation of the physicians medicine book from Latin to English so that all my fellow

countrymen and apothecaries can understand what the doctors write on their bills. Hitherto they made medicine a secret
conspiracy, writing prescriptions in mysterious Latin to hide
ignorance and to impress upon the patient.'

'You are studious as always and devoted to the art of
medicine just as you have always been since you were a boy
in Isfield. The physicians must be grateful to you that you help
them do their work,' said Elisabeth.

'No, on the contrary, I am sure they hate me and they have
never asked me to write anything for them. They want to keep
their book a secret, not for everybody to know. Not long ago
parsons, like the predecessors of grand-father, used to preach
and pray in Latin, whether he or his parishioners understood
anything of this language or not. This practice, though sacred
in the eyes of our ancestors, appears ridiculous to us. Now
everybody enjoys the gospel in plain English. I am covinced
the same must happen with medicine and prescriptions.'

'Yes, but even we ordinary people do not know when
properly to apply physick and how to prepare medicines.'

'That may be the case, but Elisabeth, think of something else,
this practice is not only ridiculous upon common sense, but it
is likewise dangerous. However capable physicians may be of
writing a prescription in Latin I am certain that some apothecaries are not always in a condition to read it, particularly
if left to an apprentice. This means that the greatest man in
the Commonwealth even when he seeks a first-rate physician,
in reality trusts his life in the hand of an idle boy. Mistakes
will sometimes happen in spite of the greatest care and skill,
but where human lives are concerned all means should be
employed to prevent them. For this reason, the prescriptions
of physicians, instead of being disguised in mystical characters
and a dead language, ought in my humble opinion, to be
conceived in the most plain and obvious terms imaginable.'[3]

'You may be right in that, but you cannot make everybody
a physician and medicine is not the same as the Gospel. God's
holy word must be taught to everyone, but medicine is not for
everybody.'

Anthony also joined the argument:

'Be careful and do not attempt an illegal translation or
anything that can harm you and your family. People in high
places may indict you before the Star-Chamber.'

'The Star-Chamber has been abolished, thank God, and I am not afraid of punishment. Imagine the doctors saying, that laying medicine more open to mankind would lessen their patient's faith in it. The truth is that opening the book also shows what jumble of obscure and costly ingredients the prescriber intends to burden our stomachs with.'[3]

'You are a fool to disregard the powerful physicians, who might accuse you of infringement on their rights, why don't you let others try?'

'I am not afraid of them, although they call me a quack, a mountebank, a deceiver, these dumb people. They do not know what they are talking about. I am not only translating the medicine book but I see it as my plight to explain the usefulness of their prescriptions and when necessary add comments about the dangers of their physick of using some chymicals and obscure mixtures of foreign herbs.'

Already as an apprentice Culpeper had been faced with the sacred Latin codex of the physicians. He had struggled with its strict directions and his critical mind often instilled rebellious thoughts about the unreasonable prescriptions which many of his fellow apothecaries hardly understood. Was it justified and should the apothecary not be allowed to think for himself?

Culpeper's idea to translate the 1618 *London Pharmacopoea* came to him as a way to prove himself, foremost towards the closed society of the privileged physicians but also to his fellow apothecaries. He was the aborted physician, who never took a university degree and who had to work hard as a simple apprentice in an apothecary shop, grinding away ingredients in a mortar, distilling, carrying supplies and running errands. He came from a genteel family with highly educated and studied members.

From the beginning of his education his mother and grandfather had destined him for a high profession and their greatest wish was that he chose divinity. In their aim they were surely not only guided by ambition but had reason to believe that he would embark on a brilliant career because of his natural gifts of intelligence and energy. When they realised that Nicholas' inclinations were not towards the spiritual calling they finally accepted that he studied medicine. But this did not materialise after the disastrous debacle with his unsuccessful elopment. In the end he did not even bother to become a free man of the Apothecary Society.

He did not fit into any of the fixed slots of society of his own family or in professional terms. Culpeper staked out his own destiny and vocation, outside the city, 'dwelling on the east-side of Spittle-fields, near London,' not a physician nor apothecary not a scientist – but to the end of his life a 'Student of Physic and Astrology.'

When Culpeper came to London in 1634 the *pharmacopoeia* or dispensatory had been enforced for only 16 years, and the former grocers and spicers were not prepared to cope with the Latin text. Culpeper as an apothecary apprentice was overqualified for his job; he had grammar school and university training in cassical languages and obviously also had attended lectures in medicine, because he was well versed with the teachings of Hippocrates and Galen. Moreover, he probably possessed a good deal of medical knowledge which he had acquired on his own, starting in his grandfather's house in Isfield.

To any apothecary who had trouble comprehending the cryptic Latin prescriptions brought from the physicians it must have been a great asset to have an apprentice who was well versed in classical languages. 'Being himself excellent in the Latine, he taught Mr. Drake in 'Threadneedle Street that tongue in less then a year and a half.'[4]

It was hinted that the translation was not a project undertaken by Culpeper on his own account. This is understandable since Culpeper among his peers probably earned the reputation of being a learned man because he could translate Latin and Greek texts his fellow apothecaries did not understand. Therefore it can be assumed that some of them encouraged him to prepare an English translation of the dispensatory.

Culpeper started working on the translation of the Latin text of the *Pharmacopoeia Londinensis* some years before it appeared 1649. It is likely that he began with handwritten bills which he distributed to his peers to help them in their work of compounding medicines according to the new Latin text.

When in 1649 Culpeper published his translation the *Pharmacopoeia* had been in use for 31 years. Culpeper's version of the *London Dispensatory* was not merely a translation from the original Latin text. Far from it, Culpeper everywhere added his own comments as to the use and virtues of each drug, quite contrary to the intention of the College of Physicians. Their president, Dr Theodor Mayerne clearly explained their intention:

In most the older, as well as the more recent antidotaria,
the use and medical attributes of each remedy have been
described. From this quiver the itinerant drug peddlers and
the quacks, being as ignorant as they are unscrupulous, equip
themselves for their medical practice, and seizing our weapons, are reponsible for the death of the sick, to the great
detriment of the state. We, therefore, do not add anything
about efficacy of the medicines. We write this book only for
the learned, for the disciples of Apollo, and for the welfare,
not for the information, of the common people. The work is
similar to that which forms the theme of the *legend of Pandora*.
Here the Gods have brought together all under their sign.[5]

This was the view of the physicians about their pharmacopoeia.
Did Pandora's box contain the gift of all, the heavenly fire
Prometheus stole from Zeus? Fire of knowledge or the cause of
the ills of mankind ? The College certainly believed in the former.

In 1649 after many pains Culpeper's translation was ready under
the title: *A Physicall Directory, or a translation of the London Dispensatory*. Culpeper felt exhausted after the intense work. In the
introductory epistle Culpeper writes: 'I am exceeding melancholy
of complexion subject to consumption and chilliness of my vital
spirit, a sickly life being alloted me in this city. God has given me
a sickly body which I am contended to wear out for my countries
good.'

When Culpeper's work appeared it immediately created a storm
of indignation. In the royalist paper *Mercurius Pragmaticus* the accusation was made:

> The Pharmacopoeia was done very filthily into English by one
> Nicholas Culpeper who commenced the several degrees of
> independency, Brownisme, Anabaptisme; admitted himself of
> John Goodwin's schoole of all ungodlinesse in Coleman Street;
> after that turned seeker, manifesterian, and now he is arrived
> at the battlement of an absolute atheist, and by two yeers
> drunken labour hath gallimawfred the apothecaries book into
> nonsense, mixing every receipt therein with some scruples, at
> least, of rebellion or atheisme, besides the danger of poisoning
> men's bodies. And to supply his drunkenness and leachery
> with a thirty shillings reward endeavoured to bring into oblo-
> quy the famous societies of apothecaries and chyrurgeons.[6]

As expected Culpeper's translation also created an outcry from
the members of the College.[6] The Physicians criticised Culpeper's
translation on the grounds that the dispensatory in the hands of
laymen might have dangerous consequences. To this Culpeper
replied:

> It being a general outcry that I do harm by instructing people
> in a way to give themselves physick. It is a wonder they will
> suffer cutlers to sell knives for fear children should cut their
> fingers and men their throats. . . . I remember a pretty fable
> in Aesop, which was like this: a nightingale and a cuckoo
> could not agree which sang the sweetest tune. The cuckoo
> pleading he did, and the nightingale pleading she did. At last
> the contention growing sharp they agreed to be tried by the
> next passenger that came by, which by accident was an ass.
> The ass said he could not judge unless he heard them both
> sing, they consented and each sung each his tune. Quoteth the
> ass: Mrs nightingale you sing very sweetly, but for a plain note
> give me the cuckoo. Alas quote the nightingale, what ill luck
> had I to be tried by an ass? I have others to make the moral. It
> is sufficient to me that my conscience tells me the thing I do is
> just. I have others to fret in their own grease, and leave mine
> own writings to the approbation or condemnation of time and
> resolve with myself to live and die a servant to my country in
> what I can with brain and pen.

The second edition of Culpeper's *A Physical Directory* appeared
in 1650. He addressed the College of Physicians: 'All your skill in
physick might have been written in the inside of a ring . . . Colledg,
colledg, thou are diseased, the cause is mammon. The diagnostics
are these: *Ipse dixit,* seven miles about London, lay him in prison:
five pound a month for practising physick unless he be a collegiate.
Be as proud as Lucifer, ride in state with a foot-cloth, love the sight
of angels (a coin), cheat the rich, neglect the poor, do nothing without
money, be self-conceited, be angry.'[7]

The College of Physicians in their criticism of Culpeper also spoke
about him as an imposter and empiric. This in a nutshell characterised the accepted view of the majority of contemporary established
physicians. They ridiculed empiricism, the name applied to a school
of thought which literally admits of nothing as true but what is
the result of experience, rejecting all *a priori* knowledge. But it is

significant that in the 17th century an 'empiric' was considered a quack; or charlatan; a pretender to medical knowledge and one who begins to practise medicine without a regular professional education of the codices of Galen and Hippocrates, relying solely on his experience and observation.

Despite these outcries it may seem surprising that no legal action was taken by the College against Culpeper. The College's monopoly and legal status had been granted by Royal charter and its members could have prosecuted Culpeper. However, times were such that it would have been difficult to try a man who always spoke in favour of the Commonwealth and the common people:

> The Liberty of the Common-Wealth . . . is most infringed by three sorts of men, priests, physitions, lawyers; . . . The one deceives men in matters belonging to their soul, the other in matters belonging to their bodies, and the third in matters belonging to their estates.

In fact, the legal privileges granted by the King were seriously threatened by social criticism which accompanied the Civil War. Monopolies, both commercial and professional, were held to be among the worst abuses of the King's government.[8]

In January of 1649, prior to the edition of the *Physical Directory*, King Charles I was executed. Therefore, it is understandable that royalist physicians could not expect much active support for their conservative ideas.

What did Culpeper's version of the Dispensatory contain? – the 1650 issue was far more than a 'National Formulary' for the standardisation of medicines, it had become a real encyclopedia of medical knowledge, not only a *verbatim* translation of the Latin text but also containing Culpeper's own comments, a 'Key to Galen and Hippocrates Art of Physick' and a chapter on some astrological speculations.[7]

It starts with a catalogue of the ingredients, 'simples' taken from the old 1618 edition. At the end Culpeper remarks: 'Thus much for the old dispensatory, which is now like an almanack out of date. Indeed had not the printer desired it might be (left out).' Then another catalogue of simples of the new dispensatory, enumerating all the ingredients: 'roots, barks, herbs, flowers, fruits, buds, seeds, tears, liquors, rosins, juices, living creatures, excrements, metals, minerals and stones.'

After that follows the long list of compound medicines with distilled water, spirits, tinctures, wines, syrups, lochochs, pouders, electuaries, oils, ointments, plasters etc. These are always presented in such a way as to tell the reader about what the official body, the 'College', says about constituents and mode of preparation; 'Culpeper' with his own comments follows, sometimes expressing disagreement with the ingredients or the way of preparation, followed by an extensive list of indications and contraindications, i.e. advice to common people how and when to use the medicine and when not (!), and finally something about the actual dosage.

This principle was quite new since for the first time it presented the public with more than a list of officinals of a National Formulary. It really was the first handbook of family medicine, akin to William Buchan's popular *Domestic Medicine* which appeared in Britain more than 100 years later.[9]

The catalogue of 'living creatures and excrements' is like a journey through a zoo or museum of natural history. Culpeper remarks: 'the College acquaints you, that there are certain living creatures called: bees, woodlice, crabs of the river, little puppy dogs, grashoppers, cantharides, cochineal, hedge-hogs, emets or ants, larks, swallows and their young ones, horse leeches, snails, earthworms, dish-washers or wagtails, house sparrows and hedge sparrows, frogs, scincus, land scorpions, moles or worms, tortise of the woods, tenches, vipers and foxes.'

Culpeper's comments: 'that part of this crew of cattle, and some others which they have not been pleased to name, may be made beneficial to your sick bodies, be pleased to understand that bees being burnt to ashes, trimly deck with hair a bald head being washed with it.'

Snails were believed to be excellent remedies for tuberculosis and the tale goes that:

> Snails with shells on their backs, being first washed from the dirt, then shells broken, and they boiled in spring water, but not scummed at all, for the scum will sink of itself, and the water drunk for ordinary drink, is a most admirable remedy for a consumption; and here, by the way, I cannot but admire at the simplicity of most physicians, who prescribe, that the snails ought to be purged from their slime either with salt or bran before they be used; which if you do, you take away their virtues: for the reason why they cure a consumption is this:

man being made of slime of the earth, the slimy substance
recovers him when he is wasted: if you please to eat the snails
when they are boiled you may, for they have a very pleasant
taste, and it would be very cunningly done of you if you did so,
especially in these hard times, for when they have meat, drink
and medicine altogether.

Snails remained a favourite cure for consumption and apparently
this was brought to North America with the early settlers; in 1929
it could still be found in the Blue Ridge Mountains where the cure
was even more drastic, in that a live snail had to be swallowed every
morning. The idea was that slime healed the lungs.[10]

'The use of fats and suets you shall have, if you please . . . the
other which you think not useful for physick, will serve to laugh at,
the reading of them may make you merry, tho' the smell of them
might turn your stomach: My self cannot chuse but smile to think in
what part the apothecaries shop the College would have them kept,
they had need place them next the civet pot.'

The second edition of 1650 contains 88 items from the animal
kingdom, compared to 33 in the first edition of 1618. It also includes
mummies from Egypt. Particularly noteworthy is the increase in
such exotic specimens as: silk-worms, cantharides (spanish fly),
cochinel (cactus insect), skink from north Africa, pardal (leopard),
viper, spermaceti and rhinoceros. This is not surprising with the
increasing overseas connections and the American and East India
trade. It also, however, reflects the importance attributed to the
magical influence of animal remedies, since it is easy to realise that
there is more magic in the animal than plant remedies, particularly if
neither the patient nor the doctor has realistic first-hand knowledge
of the strange stuff. Therefore, such medicines from exotic sources
must have had considerable suggestive power and could be excellent placebos (a placebo being an inert substance represented to be
an active drug). Under appropriate circumstances, and particularly
when anticipation is great, therapy with placebos can produce quite
striking effects. In controlled clinical trials it has repeatedly been
shown that one-third of patients will report appreciable relief from
pain following the administration of a placebo. Faith and anticipation are the cornerstones of placebo. Trust in the physician or his
remedies alone creates anticipation of a positive effect.[11]

'Chemical preparations' are briefly mentioned at the end of the
Dispensatory and describe preparations containing antinomy, iron,

sulphur, salpeter, ammoniak, mercury, lead and potassium salts. Culpeper did not think much of them and obviously he did not have any experience with such novelties since this is the only section without comments by the translator. He is only concerned with the compound preparations of 'Chemical Oils' and about the oil of vitriol he says: 'It must be mixed with other medicines' for it kills being taken alone.

In the constituents section with the heading: 'Metals, Stones, Salts and other minerals' Culpeper tells us: 'Of some precious stones I spake before in the former edition: I shall here reduce them all into order, and treat of such as were casually there omitted; wether they were mentioned by the College or not, it matters nothing to me.'

Serious promotion of chemical medicines by the College was first done by Theodore de Mayerne, who had given offence to strict Galenists by his interest in drugs such as calomel (mercurous chloride).[12]

However, in 1650, at the time of the second edition of the *London Pharmacopoeia*, chemical medicines became more and more important and Culpeper obviously makes concession to popular demand, although he feels much more comfortable with the real simples, his herbs. He does not think that the College or he, for that matter, is capable of understanding the mysteries of such novelties; they should be handled by alchemists:

> Our best way to learn to still chymical oils, is to learn of an alchymist. For I rest confident, the greatest part of the College had no more skill in chymistry than I have in building houses. But having found out certain models in old trusty authors, tell people so they must be done. I can teach a man so, how to build a house: First he may lay the foundation, then rear up the sides, then join the rafters, then build the chimneys, tile the top, and plaster the walls, but how to do one jot of this, I know not. And so play the College here, for the alchymists have a better way by far . . .

The introduction of 'chymical medicines', new medicinal products from the laboratories of alchemists at the expense of herbal drugs, was nothing less than a pharmaceutical revolution. The new 'chemical philosophy' was based on the teaching of the Swiss-German physician Paracelsus and the Belgian Van Helmont. They rejected the traditional teachings of Galen but studied nature and its elements and the 'Book of Heavens'.[13,14] One reason why Culpeper does not dismiss 'chymicals' altogether probably has to do with his astrological interests which he shared with Paracelsus.

The concept of chemical medicines admittedly in the long run paved the way for future useful inventions in pharmacology, but the type of these medicines made available at the time of Culpeper must have had devastating consequences for the well-being of patients. Certainly it was better to be stuffed with inert complex compositions of excrements, mummies and dried leaves than to be slowly poisoned by mercury, lead and oil of vitriol (sulphuric acid).

It should, however, be realised that Culpeper's favourite simple: wormwood, *'artemisia absinthium'*, is not innocuous either. The principal extract of the herb, a bitter, dark green oil, once formed the main ingredient of absinthe, an aromatic liqueur popular in France. Unfortunately, drinking absinthe was like drinking a slow-acting poison. In time it upset the nervous system, irritated the stomach and increased the action of the heart. If taken in quantity, or too often, it caused disorientation, even delirium and hallucinations. These profound mental changes are probably related to a toxic substance, thujone, which may interact with structures in the brain also activated by cannabis (ingredient of hashish). The inevitable end result was that absinthe was forbidden in France as well as the United States. Small amounts are still added to vermouth and some 'bitters'.[15,16]

Another dangerous plant is fern, or bracken, which Culpeper advocated against 'worms in the body and swelling and hardness of the spleen'. Bracken has been found to be poisonous, inhibiting the blood producing organs; it is apparently linked to cancer.[17]

In 1650 the College of Physicians issued a revised edition of the *London Pharmacopoeia*. Also translated by Culpeper it appeared in 1653 and now was offered not only to apothecaries to help them preparing medicines but to ordinary people, a trend which had more specifically been followed in his own 1652 publication, *The English Physitian* (The *Herbal*). The introduction reads: 'so that they may cure themselves, and never be beholding to such physitians as the inequity of the times affords.' The new edition contained more of his commentaries and the title-page announced that the work contained 'Three hundred useful additions'.

'Mr. Culpeper being truly sensible made it his business not to puzzle his young students with the multiplicity of medicines but only to select and set down such as are most proper choice.' This was one of the messages Culpeper had in mind when he translated the *London Pharmacopoeia*. He was not fond of polypharmacy (a medicine composed of many ingredients), particularly if they were composed of many expensive exotic simples.

It is quite typical of him that he could not abstain from adding his own comments to the catalogue of 'simples' and 'compounds'. He was particularly critical about the expensive panacea and famous antiplague drugs, the electuary of Mithridates and Venice Theriac. If he could have decided he would not have them included at all in the *London Pharmacopoeia*.

> I am loth to leave out this medicine which, if it were stretched out and cut into thongs, would reach around the world . . . Divers authors have spent more time about this and Venice treacle, both of them being terrible messes altogether, reducing them into classes, than ever they did in saying their prayers.

Theriac or treacle, from theriakos = of wild or venomous beast, was the name of a medicine used originally against poisonous bites and later as a universal remedy or panacea for particularly infectious diseases like the plague. The highest reputation had the Theriac of King Mithridates VI of Asia Minor. Later in Rome the Greek physician Andromachus added the flesh of vipers to the long list of ingredients. The three different theriacs of the *London Pharmacopoeia* contained 32 to 64 components. The 'London treacle' was wholly herbal but all theriacs contained the narcotic opium. In England it was mostly used as an analgesic and tranquilizer. It is therefore not surprising that this modification containing only nine ingredients plus opium could still be found in official pharmacopoeias until the end of the last century.[5] It is fair to say that 'Never has a medicine containing so much cured so little'.

In order to appreciate the background of Culpeper's work to print an English version of the 1618 *Pharmacopoeia Londinensis* it is necessary to briefly review a few facts about the history of medical practice in England: At the beginning of the *middle ages* there was no clear distinction between physicians, apothecaries or surgeons. One of the earliest officially acknowledged professional fraternities was that of the Barbers (1308).

The Guild of Barbers and Surgeons was officially established in 1540 by decree of Henry VIII who authorised them the supply of four executed criminals annually, a significant recognition of their anatomical experiments.[18,19]

The licence to be a physician was originally bestowed by the church and the physicians never formed a livery company. But in 1518, under Henry VIII, the College of Physicians was created. The reasons for forming the incorporation, as set forth in the original Royal charter, was: 'To check men who profess physic rather from avarice than in good faith, to the damage of credulous people. And the King founded a College of learned men.'

In the medical profession the physicians were at the top of the hierarchy, then came the barber-surgeons, the apothecaries and finally the druggists and spicers. By Act of Parliament, and as an expression of their leading role in medicine in 1540, physicians were empowered to enter the houses of the apothecaries in London to 'search, view and see the apothecary wares, drugs and stuffs and to destroy such as found corrupt or unfit for use'. Pepperers, spicers and grocers had also been suppliers of medicines but in 1607 King James I gave special privileges to the apothecaries and finally on December 6, 1618, they were recognised as fully independent. Now they could form a separate City Guild called the 'Master Wardens, and Society of the Art and Mystery of the Apothecaries of the City of London'.[20,21]

In 1618 when the new guild of apothecaries was formed it was high time for the Royal College of Physicans to finish work on unifying regulations that should govern the work of the apothecaries if the physicians wanted to maintain supremacy in their role to control the profession of medicine makers. They were supposed to be the official guide for the standardisation and formulation of medicines in England. Work on the *London Pharmacopoeia* had already started in 1585 and was conducted by a special committee of members of the College, but as it 'seemed a toilsome task' the matter was postponed until 1589 when it was again 'proposed, considered and resolved that there shall be constituted one definite public and uniform dispensatory or formulary of medical prescriptions obligatory for apothecary shops'.[22]

Whenever the text seemed ready, new concepts appeared and discussions started again about revisions. Finally on May 7, 1618, a century after its foundation, the College of Physicians edited the first edition of the London Dispensatory or *Pharmacopoeia Londinensis*.[22] A committee of 33 members had prepared the text. Among them was Theodore de Mayerne and

William Harvey, assisted by the apothecary John Parkinson, editor of two famous herbals, the *Paradisi in sole* and the *Theatrum botanicum*.

In the introduction it was pointed out that: 'For when he (King James I) granted new liberties, new privileges to the Apothecaries of London, by his letters patent, inculates upon this above all, that when the dispensatory comes out to public view they should religiously bind themselves to that as a sacred rule and should obey the decrees of the College of Physitians.'

In the Royal proclamation which followed after the introduction, King James I declared that the *Pharmacopoea Londinensis* should be enforced throughout 'Our realm of England and the Dominions thereof . . . by penalty and punishment as may be inflicted upon offenders herein.' This became the first dispensatory in the world designed for a whole nation.

Strangely enough this first issue was soon withdrawn and a new version appeared only one day after the apothecaries had received their Royal Charter, on December 7, 1618. The reason was not only typographical errors, as indicated in the preface, but rather a change of emphasis. The first issue tried to introduce simplicity in formulation and number of ingredients but this met with opposition and the final December issue was enlarged, a victory for the old principles of polypharmacy and emphasis on obscure animal ingredients. The new version included 1028 simples (simple drugs), 271 herbs, 138 roots and 138 seeds. It also contained 193 parts of animals or their excrements and 932 preparartions.

The second edition of Culpeper's translation of the *Dispensatory* was finalised in January 1653. It was based on the revised edition edition of the *Latin Pharmacopoeia* published by the College of Physicians in 1650.

The demand for the *London Dispensatory* was great and a pirate edition appeared already in 1654 by 'A Well-wisher to the Commonwealth of England'; it was reprinted fourteen times before 1718. The last edition, printed at Boston, Massachusetts, in 1720, was the second medical book after Culpeper's *Herbal* to be printed in North America (see Chapter 15).

In his endeavour to translate the *London Pharmacopoeia*, Culpeper was guided by his concern about the attitude of the College to monopolise knowledge to outsiders. According to the *statuta moralia*, revised by the College in 1647, even discussion of medical terms and treatment before patients had to be conducted in Latin. In

Culpeper's eyes, the College behaved like the pope, hiding its superstitious ignorance in a language not understood by common men.

Culpeper explained his concept:

> All the ancient physitians wrote in their own mother tongue and native language. Mesue, Avicenna, Rhaziz Serapio in Arabic, Galen and Hippocrates in Greek, Paracelsus in high dutsch. Did these do their countries good or harm think ye? What reason can be given why England should be deprived of the benefit of other nations? Worthy countrymen the College doth in effect say that you are the greatest fools under the sun.[3]

Culpeper also fought for another important idea: healing as a gift of God, that should be available to everybody and free. In the 16th and the beginning of the 17th century a physician was still mostly regarded as a wise man, a person who had been given healing power by God's grace. This can be understood as a continuation of the medieval custom of medical practice which was part of the benevolent acts of the church and convents or the expression of witchcraft. The holy act of healing was outside the sphere of trade and crafts and therefore not considered a profession that should be paid for like that of the barber or druggist. Already in 1163 Pope Alexander forbade clergy practising surgery which was not considered appropriate.

So, since healing was a gift of God to mankind, it should be free or at least not a service that one could bargain for. But although physicians were supposed to be above the mercantile aspects of their fellow health promoters, they expected to be rewarded handsomely and the gold coin (an 'angel') was a common fee.

9
Midwifery, 1651

Accuse not nature, she has done her part,
Do thou but thine.

John Milton, 1608–1674

One of the mysteries of Nicholas Culpeper's life is his great devotion to midwifery and childbirth and his obsession to describe sex organs. It is surprising that Culpeper's first own medical text two years after the translation of the *London Dispensatory* was not about herbal medicine, but about midwifery (obstetrics) and child care (pediatrics).

Culpepers new book was entitled: 'A Directory for Midwives: or a Guide for women, in their conception, bearing and suckling their children etc', and appeared on January 28, 1651. This text is a neglected and suppressed work of English Medicine which is worth resurrection because it contains a wealth of contemporary information and, not the least, it is a most enjoyable piece of English literature.[1]

Why did he deviate from his main interests: herbal medicine and astrology? No doubt this forgotten masterpiece of English medicine was born out of necessity and what must have been Culpeper's greatest frustation in life: a diseased wife and her inability to have healthy children. In the text Culpeper confesses: 'Myself having buried many of my children young, caused me to fix my thoughts intently upon this business.'

What actually was the problem? The scanty notes about Culpeper's life do not reveal anything about the mystery. Only careful studies of Culpeper's vast production gives little clues here and there, and the puzzle put together opens up a rather clear picture of what happened:

In 1640 he had married fifteen-year-old Alice Fields. During their fourteen years of marriage they produced seven children, but only the fourth, Mary, survived her father. We do not know any details about the other children, but we hear of a sick boy. This can be inferred from an incident which Culpeper relates in his *English Physitian* of 1652:

> You may remember, that not long since there was a raging disease called the bloody-flux, the College of Physicians not knowing what to make of it called it the plague of the guts, for their wits were at *ne plus ultra* about it. My son was taken ill with the same disease, and the excoriation of his bowls were exeeding great. Myself being in the country, was sent for up. The only thing I gave him was mallows bruised and boiled both in his milk and drink, in two days (the blessing of God being upon it) cured him. And here to shew my thankfulness to God, in communicating it to his creatures, leave it to posterity.[2]

Obviously at the time his boy was a little child drinking milk. Despite the medical skills of his father the poor little boy died in infancy since later there is no mention of him; we only hear Alice speaking of her surviving 'orphan' daughter Mary.

Alice Culpeper's health problem had to do with kidney disease. Nicholas lets us know about that in his treatise *'Urinalia'* where he mentions that his wife had recurrent pregnancy-related renal disease: 'My wife has with every child been extremely perplexed with this disease yet I never knew the cause of it before the writing hereof.'[3]

Pregnancy frequently results in progression of renal disease and flare-ups of chronic pyelonephritis (kidney infection). If untreated the outlook is poor both for mother and child, because gestations are frequently complicated by pregnancy hypertension or preeclampsia, a serious illness. From the description of Alice's many unsuccessful births it is very likely that she developed just that, a disease which is frequently associated with stillbirths or births of poorly developed babies with a high mortality rate. The disease is still an enigma of modern medicine for which there is no specific cure.[4,5]

Alice Culpeper died at the age of thirty-four in 1659, only five years after her husband. Culpeper, with the sad experience in his own marriage, was of the opinion that:

> No part of medicine is of more general importance than that
> which relates to the nursing and management of children.
> Yet few parents pay proper attention to it. They leave their
> tender offspring to the sole care of nurses, who are either
> too negligent to do their duty or too ignorant to know it.
> I venture to affirm that more human lives are lost by the
> carelessness and inattention of parents and nurses than are
> saved by physicians. A sensible lady therefore should read
> a medical treatise which will instruct her in the management
> of her children. A little medical knowledge about cleanliness
> and care can do more good than many costly potions from the
> apothecary.

Today the last statement seems self evident in all its simplicity,
but it was not in the seventeenth century, the age of epidemics and
mass deaths. In order to fully appreciate Culpeper's revolutionary
advice we have to realise that it was written 200 years *before*
the Hungarian obstetrician Semmelweiss introduced the modern
concept of antiseptics to combat childbed-fever.

In the seventeenth century midwifery was an art practised nearly
exclusively by women who had gained their experience through
apprenticeship and long tradition. It had not been a subject of
learned physicians who looked upon being considered a 'He-
midwife' as something below their dignity. Obstetrics therefore
received very little attention and medieval Christian opinion still
prevailed, thinking that childbirth was the result of carnal sin to be
expiated in pain as defined in Genesis III:16.[6]

Mortality for both mother and child was high because of lack
of hygiene and it was also a consequence of indifference to the
suffering of women. It is amazing to realise that instead of being
interested in developing methods to facilitate difficult labour and
delivery, the clergy and physicians had since the Middle Ages been
more occupied with the idea how to save the soul of an innocent
unborn child in distress than to help the suffering mother and her
baby. In those days it was generally believed that baptism was necessary for salvation and since it was often impossible for a weakly
or dying child to be taken to the priest there was no alternative than
to allow the midwife to baptise. Therefore it was a big issue how the
sacrament should be administered and whether parsons, vicars or
curates should be diligent in teaching the midwives how to christen
children, in time of need, according to the rules of the church.

During this time the construction of a baptismal syringe with an extended tube for intrauterine administration of water was conceived so that the unborn infant could be baptised if delivery was not forthcoming. Very little, however, was done to save the life of mother and child.[6]

Progress made in the seventeenth century was through the new trend to train midwives and to improve their knowledge. Such a change was brought about by the fact that licensing of midwives was no longer under episcopal control but now candidates had to pass three examinations before six midwives and six surgeons. The emphasis slowly shifted from aspects of moral virtue and ecclesisiastical function (baptism) to professional competence.[7]

What was the status of midwifery and obstetrics in England in the first half of the 17th century, when Culpeper lived and worked? Midwives are of ancient origin; they were the charitable and wise women (*femmes sages*) who were allowed to assist their sisters in matters of childbirth. In towns simple barber-surgeons rather than physicians helped develop obstetrics. Of these the French were more advanced than their English counterparts and in Britain obstetrics was mainly promoted by members of the emigrant Huguenot family, the Chamberlens, who became members of the guild of Barber Surgeons of London. They developed a practical obstetrical forceps in the late 1640s, but kept its design secret for several generations while profiting greatly from its use in their practice.

One of the Chamberlens, Peter (1602–1683), even for some time became a member of the College of Physicians.[8,9] In 1680 he published *The complete Midwife's practice enlarged: A full supply of such most useful and admirable secrets, which Mr. Nicholas Culpeper in his brief treatise, and other English writers in the art of midwifry, have hitherto wilfully passed by.* Obviously this meant that the Chamberlens feared the competition for readers of Culpeper's treatise.[10]

Culpeper was not a friend of the French immigrant 'she'-physicians, who had the ambition to work as obstetricians. He did not like such innovations and was of the opinion that it was not a proper job for a man. In the introduction to his 'Directory for Midwives' he wrote: 'If you make use of these rules you will find your work easie, you need not call for help of a man-midwife, which is a disparagent, not only to yourselves but also to your profession.'

In Britain operative obstetrics had hardly appeared on the scene, and even in France caesarian section was advocated purely as *ultimum refugiens* or last resort and only at the time of the mother's death. The French surgeon Guillemeau lets us know: 'Now to know certainly, and to be assured that the women has yielded up her last breath, you shall lay upon her lips, and about her nose, some light feathers; so if she breath never so little, they will fly away. And thus being assured that she is dead, the chirurgion, presently without delay, after he hath laid her belly naked, shall there make an incician, of the length of foure fingers.'

Guillemeau also relates the unsuccessful experience of the famous surgeon Ambroise Paré's attempt to deliver by section in living mothers. He was a surgeon to the French king and contemporary of Jean Riolan, the physician and anatomist whose text Culpeper later translated into English.[11]

Culpeper's *Directory for Midwives* was a totally different type of publication. It dealt more with aspects of anatomy, physiology and preventive medicine (cleanliness, diet, exercise) and much less with the art of delivery of which Culpeper cannot have had much experience. It is also obvious that Culpeper's work was in no way a copy of the French forerunner on obstetrics in England.

In every sense Culpeper's new book was exceptional. In sharp contrast to the style of the flowery and high sounding contemporary texts Culpeper is humble, down to earth and always adds some humorous or sarcastic comments. The dedication in Culpeper's *Midwifery* is moving in its simplicity and revealed something of the humble character of the author. It was not, as customary, addressed to a notable patron but 'To the matron' and read:

> If you by your experiences find anything which I have written in this book not to be according to the truth (for I am but a man and therefore subject to failings) first judge charitably of me, acquaint me with them, and they shall be both acknowledged and amended.

Furthermore he says:

> My rules are very plain and easie enough; neither are they so many that they will burden your brain, nor so few that they will be insufficient for your necessity. If you make use of them, you will find your work easie, you need not call for the help of a Man-Midwife, which is a disparagement, not only to yourselves, but also to your profession. . . . If any want

wisdom, let him ask it of God (not the College of Physitians, for if they do they may have to go without their errand, unless they bring mony with them).

The directory contains nine sections (called books). The first covers extensively 'The Instruments dedicated to Generation' (anatomy). The second is on embryology: 'Of the Formation of the Child in the Womb'. The third gives advice about questions of fertility: 'Of what hinders Conception, together with its Remedies'. The fourth chapter gives sensible advice in questions of 'What furthers Conception'. Then comes the text on pregnancy: 'A Guide for Women in Conception'. Chapter 6 and 7 are devoted to labour and miscarriage. Chapter 8 is 'A Guide for women in their lying-in' and in the final chapter we are presented with a useful treatise about the 'Nursing of Children'.

One advantage of Culpeper's *Midwifery* is the paucity of astrological speculations. There is only a short section on 'The formation of the child in the womb, astrologically handled'. In the rest of the text the reader gets the impression that astrology has nothing to do with the rational concepts of midwifery. Exercise, healthy food and cleanliness are the chief ingredients of Culpeper's advice.

Culpeper's ambition to write a manual on midwifery and child healthcare was dictated by his personal experience of his family situation. If at all possible he wanted to see a solution to his own problems and to those of others. Therefore his own quest for knowledge was matched with his ambition to be the educator of laymen and aspiring midwives. About this he writes: 'I am determined to write of the preservation of man even from conception to his grave.'[1]

His text was mainly intended to widen the horizon of the midwife by giving her a knowledge of anatomy, preventive care during pregnancy, herbal cures and child health. It was not a textbook on the craft of obstetrics and the tricks to extract a baby from the womb at difficult labour. Culpeper mostly gives information about preventive measures in 'Conception and Bearing of Children' but he does not pretend to be an expert in the art of delivery. The problems of difficult labour were the business of the surgeon, therefore he did not write about matters related to the manual skills of accouchement: 'I have not medled with your callings nor manuel operations, lest I should discover my ignorance like Phormio the philosopher, who having never seen battel, undertook to read a military lecture before Hanibal.'

As always in his writings, Culpeper asked the questions 'why' and 'how'. He started with the basic facts, the conditions of structure and function: anatomy and physiology. Culpeper was well informed about modern anatomy at a time when most authorities still believed in Galen, whose anatomical knowledge was based on dissection of monkeys and dogs.

Most of the anatomical facts presented by Culpeper are from the learned body of a large number of previously published books; he actually quotes 54 authors. It is likely that Culpeper also was influenced by Thomas Vicary's *Profitable treatise of the Anatomy of Mans Body* which he probably had already seen in his grandfather's library in Isfield.[12]

Culpeper had studied the leading anatomist of his time, Andreas Vesalius (1515–1564). He wrote: 'I would not willingly here pass by one subtil trick of Vessalius, who viewing exactly the anatomy of a bitch great with whelp (like Galen), cut the original of man in like manner. You may see it in his works for he was a publick anatomist, but he deciphered a child, not a puppy.' Culpeper also quotes *Fabricius ab Aquapendente* (1533–1619), the teacher of William Harvey.

Bookish knowledge and tradition was not enough. From his anatomical descriptions of the midwifery text we can make the amazing discovery that Culpeper, the herbalist, actually obtained first-hand knowledge about anatomy by dissection. Much of the detailed morphological descriptions were based on information obviously based on personal observations gained at *post mortem* examinations. We can conclude this because he says:

'I desire you to know that I am not unskiled in most anatomists that have written; and have been an eye witness in all I have written: my opinion is, that he is not wise that altogether neglects authors, but he is a fool in grain that believes them, before his own eyes.'

How did Culpeper, the enemy of London physicians, have access to anatomy demonstrations? Certainly not through the College of Physicians, whose prosector at that time was the famous William Harvey who held his anatomy lectures from 1615–1656.[13]

No, there was another source: the Barber-Surgeons' anatomy lectures. It was probably easier for him to make friends with the down-to-earth surgeons who did not have the same status as the physicians. They were actually the pioneers in medical education in Britain and their public 'Anatomies' had already started before the physicians' in 1546. In the text Culpeper actually mentions 'Dr. Read and some other good anatomists.'

Alexander Read (1580–1641) began anatomical demonstrations for the Barber-Surgeons in 1632.[14] Later he also became a fellow of the College of Physicians; therefore it is surprising that he was praised by Culpeper. The reason probably being that he admitted him to his demonstrations. There is another entry in Culpeper's 'Galen's Art of Physick' which indicates that Culpeper actually collaborated with surgeons to improve his anatomical knowledge: 'I was once to satisfie my mind, where a chyrurgion dissected the eye of a sheep and the eye of a cat, because we were willing to see what reason might be given why the one could see better in the night than the other; the reasons were found to be these . . . '[15]

'Another good anatomist' with the right political colour which must have suited Culpeper was Jonathan Goddard, (1617–1675) who in 1646 became lecturer in anatomy of the United Company of Barber-Surgeons. Goddard was as a skilled chemist and surgeon to the Parliamentary army. He accompanied Cromwell during his campaigns. It is therefore quite likely that Culpeper attended anatomy demonstrations in the Anatomy Theatre designed by Inigo Jones and modelled on the famous anatomy theatre at Padua.[14] Goddard, however, had no high opinion about his pupil. This implies that Culpeper was not treated sympathetically by the rulers of the Commonwealth and Culpeper himself does not praise Cromwell either.

As mentioned earlier we can infer that Culpeper did not participate in Harvey's anatomy demonstrations since there is not the slightest indication that he was impressed by the new concept of the circulation of blood. Dr. Read did not believe in Harvey's teachings, so if he was Culpeper's mentor in anatomy he would not have taught him about the new concept of the circulation.[13] When we listen to Culpeper's description of spermiogenesis it becomes quite clear that he is not a pupil of Harvey's when he says:

> The Liver is the original of blood, and distributes it through the body by the veins, and not the heart, as Aristotles waking dream was . . . The heart is the original of the vital or quickening spirit, which it distributes to the body by the arteries. . the preparing veins and arteries, the one carrying blood, the other vital spirits, all tendinq to the propagation of man; all four tend down directly to the stones . . . they serve as

laborers to carry the stones what they need; as laborers carry bricks and morter to masons to build an house, so these carry blood and vital spirits to the stones to make seed, and now you know whereof seed is made, viz vital and natural blood, or blood and vital spirit (which you please) concocted by the stones.

In addition to his attendance at 'human anatomies' with a surgeon he also made his own observations in dogs. He writes about the *plexus pampiniformis*: 'these vessels make a most curious implication, intertexture. Sometimes the veins go into the arteries, sometimes the arteries into the veins, then they separate again, the beholding of which brings an exceeding deal of delight to the eye, and content the mind (I could show it any man in the anatomy of the dog.)'[1]

One of the objectives of the new text was to clarify the anatomy of the reproductive organs before he gave advice to midwives. He explains:

> I began first at the principles, namely the anatomy of the vessels dedicated to generation; for all things I hold it most fitting, that women (especially midwives) should be well skilled in the exact knowledge of the anatomy of these parts. Let it not be objected to me, that many good midwives are ignorant of it . . . A midwife is (or else should be) natures helper; and how can any help nature and not well skilled in the tools by which nature doth her work; this is the business of the book, viz to give you a brief, yet very perfect anatomy, of those members which nature useth as instruments to beget its like, to which I have added some means how to preserve them clean and pure, the neglect of which I conceive the reason of most miscarriages in women, nay and of the death of most children in their infancy . . . I have been as plain as I can, and that satisfies me, and so I hope it will do al honest poeple.

In the first book about the 'Genitals of Men' he teaches us: 'The Latins have invented very many names for the yard, I suppose done by venerious people (Which Rome it seems was full of them, since which times, vices have encreased there faster than virtues) I intend not to spend time in rehearsing the names, and as little about it's form and situation, which are both well known, it being the least part of my intent to tell people what they know, but teach them what they know not . . . The muscles of the yard are four, two on each side, and their use is to erect the yard and make it stand, and are therefore called erector.'

After he finishes his treatise about 'The Genitals of Men' he goes on to say: 'Having served my own sex, I shall see now if I can please the women, who have no more cause than men (that I know of) to be ashamed of what they have, and would be grieved (as they had cause, for they could not live), if they were without, but have cause if they rightly consider of it, to thank me for telling them something they know not.'

When he starts with 'The Privy Passage' quite some space is devoted to the hymen: 'a thin and sinewy skin . . . a certain note of virginity where ever it is found, for the first act of copulation breaks it. I confess much controversie has been among anatomists concerning this, some holding there is no such thing at all, others that it is but very rare; the truth is, most virgins have it, some hold all, I must suspend my own judgment til more years brings me more experience: yet this is certain, it may be broken without copulation, as it may be gnawn asunder by defluxion of sharp humors, especially in young virgins, because it is thinnest in them, as also by unskilful applying pessaries to provoke the terms, and how many ways God knows.'

Then he continues to quote eight different anatomical authorities, in essence meaning that Roman and French anatomists hardly saw such a thing because their specimens had been obtained from 'amoral wenches', whereas 'Hebrew virgins were more chary in preserving it'.

Among others he quotes Pineaus (1550–1619) royal Parisian physician whose books on gynaecology and obstetrics often were confiscated because of the frank discussion of virginity and its method of loss.[11] Culpeper's frank description of sexual organs was not without risk, particularly in Puritan England; even in Stuart England it could be a problem to be frank about the anatomical descriptions of sex organs, certainly if presented in plain English. This happened in 1614 when the College of Physicians was seriously disturbed by the intention of Dr. Helkiah Crooke to describe human generative organs in an anatomical treatise.[13]

We must admire Culpeper for his female anatomy, particularly his view about the role of the ovaries as sources of the human egg. In many ways he was a pioneer, he did not blindly believe in old

authorities and he made his own research: 'I commit my writing to
the trial and censure of time and shall with gladness embrace that
man that in the spirit of meekness (which is next to the spirit of
God) tells me of my errors. God and good men hate idle men and
women and that you shall be methodically diligent.'

When Culpeper wrote his anatomical description he obviously
had no high opinion of Greek authors: 'I weigh not a rush the nice
definition of Aristotle and the Peripatics nor of all the fools that
dance after their pipes.' He had gathered first sight experience of
the female body from human dissections. This was not an easy task
since public dissections or 'anatomies' were reserved for physicians.
But Culpeper obviously had seen the ovaries with his own eyes
when he writes:

> Now to the business, the testicles or stones of a woman are
> for generation of seed where many times you might see in
> anatomy, (if the doctors and chyrurgions were not high base
> and denied you admittance), white thick and well concocted.
> In the act of copulation the woman spends her seed as well as
> the man, and both are united to make conception. The seed of
> both sexes being united, the womb instantly shuts up, partly
> to hinder the extamission or passing out of the seed, partly to
> cherich the seed by its inbred heat, the better to provoke it to
> action.[1]

Culpeper's view on conception was radical: he claimed that
the woman contributed with an egg. Conventional theory, even
embraced by Harvey, only attributed a passive role to the female,
receiving and nurturing the origin of life: the male semen. Before
the use of the microscope Culpeper anticipated the existence of the
female egg: 'Women have a twofold spermatical matter, the one
watery, which moistens and refreshes the womb and fruit in it, the
other which is *thick in the tubae* (the egg) which is mixed with the
seed of man to make conception.'

Straightforward and without the caution of the great scientist
Harvey, he makes his point: 'The use of the stones in women, is
the same that they are in men, viz. to concoct seed.'

Culpeper was lucky in his guess, since it is hard to believe that
he arrived at this conclusions by searching experimentation (like
Harvey's inconclusive studies on deer). But his description of the
events is as good as any during the period before Leeuvenhoek,

who in the 1660s introduced the microscope for the study of living cells. This finally made it possible to demonstrate the ovum, and it remained for the Dutch anatomist Reinier de Graaf to show the process of ovulation.

William Harvey's famous book on embryology, *Exercitationes de generatione animalium* is a lengthy experimental treatise mainly addressing the unsolved question of the development of the embryo. It is surprising to note that Harvey was never convinced about the role of an ovum supplied by the female, which is clear from this publication and the previous accounts of his anatomical lectures. Harvey put forward the then generally accepted theory of Aristotle that the male introduces the semen but the female provides nothing to the foetus except the uterus where it is to grow. Harvey did not discover the egg as a product of the ovaries. Nevertheless he coined the phrase: *omne vivum ex ovo*.[16]

Culpeper really had revolutionary ideas, not only about politics and education of the common people but also about such modern trends as physical fitness through exercise. Exercise even for young women is something he advocates:

> That ever God ordained men or women should live idly, I never yet read or heard. Lysurgus that famous Spartan commander, being asked the reason why he forced young virgins to labour answered very wisely and discreetely, that thereby cleansing their bodies of evil excrements, they might bring forth lusty children when they were married. A prudent speech well beseeming the man that uttered it, and very fit to be practised in every Commonwealth. But that I may shew how the exercise of the body of the parent conduceth to the life of the child consider: It stirs up natural heat in them. Moderate exercise equally disturbs the spirits throughout the body. The more equally your spirits are distributed in your bodies, the more equally will they be distributed in your seed; and by consequence so much more probable are your children to live. Moderate exercise by opening the pores, cleanseth the blood of those fuliginous or sooty vapours which usually offends it, and this is the reason sweating is such a good remedy in fevers. – You see, nay you cannot see, unless you are wilfully blind, that poor people such as work hard, and fare hard, and are seldom idle, have more children and those stronger and lustier of body, and usually longer lived than such that live idly.

Poor Alice with all her stillbirths! Nicholas probably forced her to run and sweat !

'Of the signs of conception' we hear a rather fancy tale:

> If she keep the seed, it is a sign she has conceived, and a man may know that his seed is kept, if he find in copulation that his yard is sucked and drawn by the womb, and the privities are not moist. And if she perceives little or no seed to come forth again, and grow chill and quiver, and perceive a twitching in her womb, from the great delight; and the mouth of the womb closeth, and the terms stop. But they are deceived when they count or reckon from the stoppage of the terms for some have their terms twice or thrice after they have conceived. The chiefest sign of conception is, when there is at first loathing of meat, pewking, pica or preternal appetite and vomiting. And when they hate that they earnestly affected, or faint when they think of them.[1]

About the question of abortion he did not hesitate with his answer: 'Wether it is lawful to cause an abortion to preserve the mother? A Christian may not cause an abortion for any cause, for it is wicked, and the gentiles in Hippocrates' time never allowed it.'

The charm of Culpeper's writings is his very special personal style and as we have seen, personal experience often initiated Culpeper's interest in studies on certain subjects, like obstetrics and gynaecology. Another exemple of this is urology. One of his children had urinary problems (probably a urinary tract infection) because he tells us: 'My own child being annoyed with one of the diseases about the year 1645 made me set out and fix my studies upon this subject.'[17]

Culpeper's writings are full of quirks and practical jokes. Therefore it is sometimes difficult to know if he is serious about certain things. One example is when he tells us how to cut the umbilical cord in boys and girls:

> The navell must be tyed longer, or shorter, according to the difference of the sexe, allowing more measure to the males: because this length doth make their tongue, and privy membres longer: whereby they may both speake the plainer, and be more serviceable to ladies. And by tying it short, and almost close to the belly in females, their tongue is lesse free,

and their naturall part more straite: and to speake the truth, the gossips commonly say merrily to the midwife; 'If it be a boy make him good measure; but if it be a wench, tye it short.'

Culpeper's style always reveals his wit and sense of humour and here and there he interjects little stories:

A certain man of ingenious breeding, and good wit (whose name I have forgotten), had a wife, whose insatiable desire could not be satisfied for want of a boy, though she had many daughters, beautiful of person, of excellent understanding, and good conditions, but a boy she must have, or else she died. To answer her distempers, (I cannot say her prayers) God gave her a boy, and he proved a fool. Said her husband to her: Wife, thou wast never contented til thou hadst a boy, and now thou hast gotten one that wil be a boy all daies of his life.

And at the end:

Blame not me for not making a long narrative how a nurse should use her child, and how she should dress its head, and how she should pin it up in blankets, and how she should hold it out to piss: let but my former rules be observed and the labor of the woman will be easie; her lying in short; her children usualy maintained in health and strength: I hope they will not blame me for shortness, unless they love long things.

As we have seen, Culpeper's *Midwifery* is not limited to issues of procreation and obstetrics, it also adresses important gynaecological problems and is one of the earliest texts on pediatrics. His *Midwifery* contains chapters on child-care and a later edition of his *Directory for Midwives* incorporated a 39-page treatise 'Cure of Infants', which expressed his concern for children and provided the first description of laryngeal spasm, simple medications and sensible advice to mothers:

A child new born sleeps more than he wakes, because his brain is very moist, and he used to sleep in the womb. If you cannot make him sleep by singing or rocking, nor the like, it is a disease. If it be from a fever or pain, remove them. Sleeping

medicines are not safe, but hurt, but are rather to be given the
nurse moderately, as sweet almonds, lettice, poppy-seeds. Coll
not the head too much, nor use narcotics. These are safe: oyl of
dill to the temples.

Another example:

'Of diet and government of newborn infants: let it sleep long,
carried in the arms often, and give it the suck, but fill not too
much his stomach with milk. It is best to wean in the spring
or fall, in the increase of the moon, and give but very little
wine.' – And later about children: 'Keep them from passions,
sorrow and fear; and cocker them not, but keep them to reason.
Let them play to temper the affection, but as not to hurt the
body.'

About nurses:

The blood that nourishes the child in the womb, is turned
into milk to nourish him after he is born, because he can
eat no solid meats. And because from weakness or disease,
the mother cannot suckle her child, she must have a nurse of
good habit of body, and red complexion, which is the sign of
the best temper; and let her not differ much from the temper
of the mother, unless it be for the better; let her be between
twenty and thirty, well bred and peaceable, not angry, not
melancholy, or foolish; not letcherous, nor a drunkard. Let
it not be after her first child, and let not her milk be too old
or too new, of ten months old at the most. Let her breasts be
well fashioned with good nipples, that the child may take them
with pleasure. Let her keep a good diet, and abstain from hard
wine and copulation, and passions; these chiefly trouble the
milk, and bring diseases upon the child.

Before the advent of baby-formulas wet nurses were a convenient
solution for many who could afford such a luxury. Culpeper is
aware of this and gives his opinion about the matter:

Question: wether is an infant better nourished by the mother
or by a nurse? Some say by a nurse; others say, the mothers
milk is more like the nourishment it had in the womb, which

is best, except she has a disease. For he that gave her strength to conceive, travel, and bring forth, will give her strength to play the nurse, though she be weak. And honest women will be very obedient to directions, for the good of the child they love so dearly.

There is an entertaining section on fertility:

Women 14–45, but young men that marry women surmounting that age aforesaid, if they expect children, unless by miracle, must labour against the wind; though if an old man that is not worn out by diseases and incontinuency, marry a brisk lively lass, there is hopes even to threescore and ten, and some that are extraordinary lusty, till forescore. Hippocrates that famous and learned physician is of the opinion that youth at 16 years or between that and 17 having much vital strength, may be capable of getting children, and that force and heat of procreation matter continually increases till 45, 50 and 65. And at the latter begins to flag, the seed by little and little becoming unfruitful, the natural spirits being extinguished and the humours dried up. 'Tis reported by a credible author that in the reign of Erecus, King of Sweedland, a man was married at a hundred years old to a bride of thirty, and had many children by her, but looked so fresh, that as knew him not took him exceed half that age.[1]

Culpeper had a fair knowledge of veneral diseases. He is well aware of the infectious nature of genital warts and syphilis, a fact that at the time was not yet generally realised. Most texts only speak about 'sharp corrupting humours'. We read about 'pustules and condyloma of the privities' and are taught that they are 'usually found in the privities and fundament of such that have the French-Pox. They are stubborn, long and infectious to men, and hard to be cured.' And also of 'cancer of the womb: it is seldom seen, and never cured; but here I shall speak of that in the neck of the womb, which is ulcerated, or not ulcerated.'

Culpeper's idea about infectious agents and immunity is revealing:

There are epidemical fevers at certain times. The cause is not only from impurity of the terms (humours), but from the malignity of the air. Sometimes it is infectious, and the humours are so corrupt, that worms breed under the scabs, and corrode the bones and internal parts, as has been seen in bodies opened, dead of this disease. If the disease is very infectious, before there is a fever, it is good to preserve by change of air and antidotes, when many dye of it; but when few dye, it is not amiss to let them alone, lest they have it in a more dangerous time, for most will have it.

This means he realised the importance of a previous not too dangerous infection for immunity.

In Culpeper's time it was not known that the plague was transmitted by fleas but by breathing foul emanations from those afflicted. Therefore fumigation by fires and perfumes was very popular. The state of hygiene was bad, particularly in the cities. Cleanliness was wanting in all aspects of life. The vivid picture drawn by the admiralty official Samuel Pepys in his famous diary clearly shows that lice were not uncommon even in better homes, and the delightful love poem of John Donne (1571–1631) about the flea is very revealing:

Marke but this flea, and marke in this,
How little that which thou deny'st me is;
It suck'd me first, and now sucks thee,
And in this flea, our two bloods mingled bee;
Thou know'st that this cannot be said
A sinn, nor shame, nor losse of maidenhead,
    Yet this enjoys before it wooe,
    And pamper'd swells with one blood made of two,
    And this, alas, is more then wee would doe.

Culpeper tells us: 'In places where bathing of children is used, let it be washed twice a week, from the seventh month, till it be weaned.' He confesses that lice are a problem in children:

Lice are creatures which bread in cloaths that are constantly worn, but they are chiefly in children from the excrements of the head. All say thet filth and nastiness alone is the cause of lice; but I think not for filth alone cannot do it without heat, for besides the first qualities, there is a hidden force in the matter by which it is disposed to produce a particular species; for fleas and worms will not breed of that matter which breeds lice; so it

is in plants . . . It is a filthy troublesome disease, many have
them breed all over the body and some have died by them.
Sometimes the lice leave them when they are about to die.
To prevent breeding lice, let children eat no food of evil juyce,
especially figs; let the head be often combed and washed.

Obstetrics and gynaecology like other branches of medicine were
dominated by the Galenic principles of temperatures and humours,
as was the conception of, and generation, of babies. In *Galen's Art of
Physick* Culpeper relates these ideas to us:

The indications of a cold and moist temperature of the testicles
are smoothness and moisture about these parts. Verseness to
the sport of Venus, they care not wether they came to that
school or not. The seed is thin, watery, unfruitful, and either
produces no conception at all or else but a weakly sickly puny
little girl at the best. Signs of hot and dry temperature of the
testicles: The seed procreative of such people is hot, dry and
thick, yet most fruitful and engenders usually the strongest
children. They are prone to venery and are offended with
compulsion to that sport.

Culpeper's comments to this are: 'If you perceive too much heat in
those parts use cooling herbs as endive, succory, lettice, plantane,
water lillies, cucumbers, melons, poppies . . . A hot and moist
womb is very fruitful, if the man be well tempered; and though
he be old and weak, yet she will conceive by him. Sometimes they
have twins, or over-do and have a mole.'
In the section about 'What furthers Conception' Culpeper says:

This I shall deliver to you by way of caution. Use not the
act of copulation too often. Some say, it makes the womb
flippery, I rather think it makes the womb more willing
to open then to shut; satiety gluts the womb, and makes
it unfit to do its office, and that's the reason why whores
have so seldom children; and also why women after long
absence of their husbands, when they come again, usually soon
conceive . . . Apish ways of copulation hinder conception.

Apart from such oddities Culpeper gives good advice. About the
right time of delivery he says:

This is what the midwives call the water and when they see that come away, then they say to them that stand by, now the birth is near, and 'tis very true, and the certainst sign that can be; for the child is no better able long to subsist in the womb after those skins are broken, than a naked man is in a heap of snow. These waters, if the child come presently after them, facilitate the labor, by making the passage slippry; and therefore let no midwives endeavor with their nails, or anything else, to force the water away. (If midwives wil force it away, let them pare their nails first, for musicians and midwives must not wear their nails too long). Dame Nature knows when the true time of birth is, better than they, and usually retains the water til that time . . . Let midwives be ruled by me, never to force away a child unless they are confident it be dead or the women laboring with it, be troubled with an immoderate flux of blood, or have convulsions.

Culpeper also writes about 'Diseases of the nipples' and advocates the help of pet dogs: 'They are either wanting, or lie hid one or both, which hinders giving suck. When they come forth first, use a sucking instrument, and then apply puppy dogs to suck.'

'The clefts in the nipples is an usual evil, and causeth great great pain in nurses; and if it continue long, it turns to foul ulcers, that they cannot give suck.' For this he gives a recipe of alum water and a metal cover which goes back to the time of the French surgeon Ambroise Paré.[18]

About stagnant milk and mastitis: 'if it stay long in the breasts, the thin evaporates, and the thick remains, and hardens to kernels, hence are hard tumors, because the cheesie part of the milk is apt to harden. If curdled milk be strong in the breats, it easily turns to an imposthume and inflammation. To hinder curdling: take powder of mints, coriander-seed each two ounces; oyl of dill an ounce; with wax make a liniment.'

We should not be deceived to believe that Culpeper only advocated gentle cures of nature and exclusively resorted to herbal remedies. No, he also sometimes, though very rarely, gives advice about bleeding and cupping. In the chapter dealing with 'Inflammation of the womb' he accepts Galen and writes:

'An erysipelas in a woman (= streptococcal infection) with child is deadly because there is an abortion, and the mother dies. The worse the symptoms, the greater the danger. And it is safer to discuss an inflammation than to ripen it: If it turns scirrus, it is lasting, and makes a dropsie. If it be not after abortion or flux of blood, open the vein of the arm, or cup and sacrifice the shoulders. Bleed not in the foot, lest you draw blood more to the womb.' – As to bleeding for disorders of the uterus Culpeper says this: 'What veins must be opened when terms are stopped? Authors disagree in this as Aetius and Galen who always speaks of the ankle-veins: and most are of his mind, being it is rational. For a vein opened in the arm, doth rather revel from the womb, then draw the blood to it. But in the ankle brings it to its place, and opens obstructions, and doth both lessen and bring blood to the womb, and move that which is in the womb fixed.'[1]

A very popular book which competed with Culpeper's 'Directory for midwifes' was *Aristotle's compleat Masterpiece*. It appeared in the 17th century and dealt with information about the structure and function of the female body, conception and childbirth. It was a compilation on the fringe of medicine attributed to Aristotle. As such one might wonder if Culpeper used this text as a source for his own text. Exactly when and where *Aristotle's compleat Masterpiece* originated is obscure although the oldest copy was supposedly found in 1694.[19] Therefore, and also because of dissimilarities of contents, it is very unlikely to have been a source for Culpeper.

As the frontispiece it displayed a nude woman in a library with attributes of learning such as books, a globe and a stuffed crocodile, standing before a man dressed as a scholar. Rather than being a textbook for midwives it was an obscure undercover publication and sex handbook containing titillating information about the 'facts of life' and as such it later became a Victorian bestseller which was issued until the 1930s.[19] It contains information similar to other 'books of knowledge', e.g. with the view that contraception is possible by copulating barefoot because the 'vital spirits' will rush down from the testes to warm the cold feet.

Culpeper's *Directory for midwives* became a bestseller and after 1651 another 17 editions appeared until 1777. The reason for this success probably partly had to do with the fact that these books, initially intended for the instruction of midwives, were exploited as a handy miniature publication and popular source of information on sexual matters and childbirth. The first editions appeared in *octavo* size, comparable to modern pocket books. Later they were reduced even further to *duodecimos*, the size of the book of Common Prayer or small Bibles.

Seventeenth-century printing was a messy affair with no rules of fair play. Anything could be copied indiscriminately. It is ironic that after his death Culpeper's text became assimilated into a multi-author textbook *The Complete Midwife's Practice* together with his original opponents, King Charles I's personal physician and president of the Royal Society of Medicine, Sir Theodore Mayerne, J. Chamberlaine, obstetrician and the French midwife, madame Louise Burgerois, as authors. The book was printed in 1680 by Obdiah Blagrave. The strangest fact, however, is that it was based on a book with the identical title *The Complete Midwife's Practice* published in 1656 by three anonymous authors: T.C., I.D., M.S. and T.B. and printed by one of Culpeper's stationers, Nathanial Brook. In essence it was stolen from Culpeper. Despite that the authors in the preface try to discriminate his work: 'A miracle to us that Mr. Culpeper, a man whom we otherwise respect should descend so low as to borrow his imperfect treatise from the wretched volumes (The Birth of Man, Child birth, The Expert midwife) and we medeal faithfully with you, that the small piece of his intituled: The Directory for Midwives, is the most desperately defficient of them all. Except he writ it for necessity, he could certainly have never been so sinfull to have exposed it to the light.'[20]

Culpeper's *Directory for Midwives* was a novelty and the first truly English textbook of its kind. The first publication in English on the subject had appeared in 1540 and was entitled: 'The birth of Mankynde' a translation from Latin of Roesslin's work: *De partu hominis*, published in Frankfurt (1532). Another one was: 'The expert midwife', a translation of *De conceptu et generatione hominis* (1554). Finally there was the translation of Guillemeau's *Childbirth, or happy delivery of women*, which appeared in 1612.[21] An eminently suitable publication, it contained all kinds of practical information primarily for surgeons and midwives; the book was illustrated with pictures of the fetus in utero, including twins and it also, displayed simple surgical instruments such as hooks. It addressed all kinds of obstetrical problems and offered rational advice e.g. in the case of ecclampsia (convulsions of pregnancy). The text concentrated on the surgical aspects of obstetrics and blood letting. Such an approach is understandable because Gillemeau was a pupil of the famous French surgeon Ambroise Paré.

The *Directory for Midwives* preceded the 1668 treatise by the French surgeon Francois Mauriceau: *The diseases of women with child, and in child bed*, translated by by Hugh Chamberlene.[11,22]

The anatomical details of Culpeper's work were largely derived from Adrian van der Spieghel's *Opera omnia* and Johannes Riolanus *Enschiridium anatomicum et pathologicum*. In later editions of Culpeper's *Midwifery*, as illustration, a plate from Spieghel was printed showing a baby attached with its umbilical cord to the placenta and displayed on the cut open amnionic layers. The picture is usually reproduced in different versions, some only showing the baby. The text owes credit to the text of Riolan which Culpeper later translated into English.

Despite these sources Culpeper's *Directory for Midwives* certainly stands out as a very original work of its own which clearly bears the stamp of its author, particularly in the therapeutic sections. It is no doubt the first English textbook on obstetrics, gynaecology and childcare.

In 1656 the *Directory for Midwives* appeared again in a revised version, this time with five brass plate illustrations taken from the anatomy books of Veslingius and Spigelius, translated by Culpeper. Although this edition appeared after Culpeper's death, it is very likely that the new material such as the illustrations by Veslingius and Spigelius were already prepared during Culpeper's lifetime since his translation of Vesling's work, entitled *The Anatomy of the Body of Man*, already appeared in 1653.[23]

In all his books we find that Culpeper wants to be as comprehensive and exhaustive as possible; we can feel his ambition to cover the whole subject like an encyclopedia. He writes: 'And this may be done methodically, for things look best when they are in order, because God is the God of order.' Culpeper was proud of his work and when finished he wrote: 'I have viewed over this work and acknowledge it as my own child.'

The College of Physicians did not welcome the book about midwifery by the troublemaker Culpeper particularly since his text is full of cynical criticism of the College:

> I cannot account it tedious, because it conduceth to the teaching of knowledge to my country men and women, who have been too long reined in with the bridle of ignorance by physicians, so that they may be better ridden by them, for just for all the world as the popish priests serve those they call

the laity, . . . so do our physicians serve the communality of
this nation. They cry out against me for writing in my mother
tongue, they bring, no other arguments than what the papists
bring for themselves. One holds the word of God, the other
physick to be a mystery, and the vulgar must be ignorant in
them both.

In the 'Conclusions' , Culpeper said: 'The remainder of my life
have I consecrated to the publick good; I expect no reward for
doing my duty; yet am forced to leave the child newly weaned,
to go upon another physical employment of public concernments.
I should very shortly take him up where I left him, and trace him
through his childhood, youth, man-hood old age, even to his grave,
where he and I shall rest in hope of Resurrection.'[24]

In his *English Midwives* Aveling in 1872 alluded to Culpeper,
'Student in Physic and Astrologie', as a 'clever, canting charlatan'
and said his book was 'despicable, barren of all useful information'.
He, however, praises the learned Drs William Harvey, Percival
Willughby and William Sermon and says: 'Independently of their
genius and learning, it will be observed that these self-constituted
instructors of midwives were men of high social standing and
medical position.' Obviously a very biased judgment not based on
facts. [25]

Harvey's book on embryology: *Exercitationes de generatione animalium*, published in Amsterdam in 1651 and later in London (1653)
also contained a section on obstetrics. This part is philosophical
and highly speculative. Harvey promotes the idea that parturition
is largely based on the activity of the foetus:

How much the foetus contributes to the acceleration and
facilitation of its own birth is plainly to be seen in the hatching
of oviparous creatures, for it is apparent that the foetus itself
breaks the eggshell and not its mother. And so it is also probable that in the birth of viviparous creatures the chief cause
of being born must be attributed to the foetus itself and to
his own endeavours . . . the foetus itself with its head turned
downward, approaches the gates of the womb and opens them
by its own strength and struggles out into the light.[16]

This misconception could have serious implications to mother and
child in delayed labour: the midwife could wrongly judge that the

foetus was 'not strong enough' to be born and this could provoke the use of cruel cutting instruments such as the apertorium and hooks to extract the baby.[26]

When considering these facts I think it is hardly justified to call Harvey 'The father of English midwifery'.[13,26] Such an epithet should more appropriately be applied to Peter Chamberlene with his vast experience and interest in the technique of delivery or to Nicholas Culpeper, who did not question the active role of the female in the process of procreation. Next to the *Herbal*, the *Midwifery* was Culpeper's most popular book; it was reprinted 17 times, the last edition in 1777.[23] From the purely medical point of view it can be considered Culpeper's most important publication, which must have had great impact on contemporary English obstetrics and child care. Culpeper is the first English physician to realise the importance of human reproductive biology. If anybody deserves to be called 'Father of English Obstetrics' or midwifery, it should be the physician from Spitalfields.

10

The Herbal, 1652

Of plants:

> 'No concoction of apothecaries can equal their excellent
> virtue. The delight is great but the use greater, and joined
> often with necessity.'
>
> John Gerard, 1545–1612

> 'The study of herbs and plants is not onely pleasant, but
> profitable, by comforting the minde, spirits, and senses
> with an harmlesse delight, and by enabling the judgment
> to confer and apply help to many dangerous diseases.'
>
> John Parkinson, 1567–1650

Samuel Leadbetter, his old apothecary friend, often visited Culpeper. Lately Nicholas had shown signs of strain. He was like a woman in labour; he wanted to complete his new book, *The English Physitian*. One week later Samuel came again. He was worried about his friend, went upstairs and said:

> 'What have you been doing all week, do you feel better,
> more cheerful than before?'
>
> 'I have been sitting up late and writing to the light of a
> candle and I have nearly finished my book of physic, my last
> will and testament. It contains the best I can give my children
> and fellow countrymen. He that reads this, and understands
> what he reads, hath a jewel of more worth than a diamond.
> There lies a key in these words which will unlock (if it be
> turned by a wise hand) the cabinet of physisk. I have delivered
> it as plain as I can; it is not only upon wormwood I wrote, but

on all plants, trees and herbs. He that understands it is not unfit in my opinion to give physick. This shall live when I am dead. And thus I leave it to the world, not caring a farthin wether they like it or dislike it. The grave equals all men, and therefore shall equal me with all princes: until which time the eternal Providence is over me. Then the ill tongue of a prating fellow, or one that has more tongue than wit, or is more proud than honest, shall never trouble me. Wisdom is justified by her children.'[1]

The next day when Peter Cole, his publisher, came to see him he said:

I have written down all my experience from healing with my own medicines. It really is so simple, but that is why it not will be approved by our physicians. I do not hesitate to say that it is part of kitchen medicine, part testimonials of others and partly my own inventions put into the frame of astrological reasoning which makes everything logical to the mind. I can deduct the virtues of simples from their appearance and influence by planets.

Culpeper was very proud of his work. It was really his own work and not a mere translation. Samuel Leadbetter was the first to receive a copy of Culpeper's new book, *The English Physitian*, which had just come fresh from the press.
Samuel was impressed:

This is a masterpiece and more than an apothecary book. It shows that you are a doctor with a new vision about healing and a book dedicated to the people of our Commonwealth, but why do you have to add all these astrological comments, why do you call it an astro-physical discourse of the vulgar herbs of this nation? You should call it the English Herbal. You are so learned and illuminated, I never understood this part of you! And how can you reconcile astrology and medicine? It cannot be denied that many men by their own industry have contradicted their stars and triumphed over the heavens, because of their own wisdom and virtue. Also some persons borne under good stars and unto good fortunes have come short of their destinie.

I cannot deny that although the heavens work by their
hidden power and influence, proclivities and inclinations,
yet they are variously alterable according to education and
circumstance and therefore affecting the power of the heavens.
No man can be denied free arbitrary choice to do or not to do,
to like or dislike. Heavenly influences are present but do not
force men's actions.

There are nativities for good haps, for ill haps, success,
losses, fortunate and unfortunate events. He who has common
sense and reason and can think will easily discover their
falsehood.

To this Culpeper replied:

But I wanted to give reasons for what I do, not like the
physitians who for want of speculation makes themselves
slaves to tradition, and tradition is the father of errors.

Invisible things are clearly seen from the creation of the
world. Friends and country men will no longer be deceived,
they will be able to study the stars which priests tell you are
conjuration and witchcraft. These priests spend whole daies,
nay weeks in rayling and scolding and writing against those
that observe them. The Lord be merciful to them, and turn
their hearts if it be his will. There are so many signs to teach
you what God is, and the stars declare their power to you.
David a man after Gods own heart admired them, as revealed
in Psalm 8, 3.4 and so do all men of David's spirit and they
that despise them shall hereafter have time enough to repent
at leasure.[2]

Culpeper acted in good faith, he was convinced he had God
on his side when he mixed astrology and medicine. By 'speculation' obviously Culpeper did not mean ideas out of the blue but
according to him it was the result of careful studies of astral forces
ordained by God. He accused the orthodox members of the church
who maintained that it was superstition.

Culpeper's *magnum opus*, and best known work to this day, the
celebrated *Herbal* appeared on November 6, 1652 and was called:
'The English Physitian, or an Astro-Physical Discourse of the Vulgar
Herbs of this Nation. Being a compleat Method of Physick, whereby
a man may preserve his Body in Health; or cure himself, being sick,

for three pence charge, with such things only as grow in England, they being most fit for English Bodies.'

The book starts with an introduction: 'To the Reader', here Culpeper in general terms tries to explain the wisdom of God and nature. He refers to the important authors who helped him write his own book and gives them credit for their work. He mentions the ancients and goes on to comment about English authors:

> In this art the worthies of our Nation, Gerard, Johnson and Parkinson are not to be forgotten, who did much good in the studie of this art, yet they and all others that wrote of the nature of herbs, gave not a bit of a reason why such an herb was appropriated to such a part of the body, nor why it cured such a diseases. Truly my own body being sickly brought me easily into a capacity to know that health was the greatest of all earthly blessings, and truly he was never sick that does not believe it. Then I considered that all medicines were compounded of herbs, roots, flowers, seeds etc. and this first set me awork in studying nature of simples . . . I always found the disease vary according to various motion of the stars . . . What remains but you labor to glorifie God and do good to yourselves first by increasing your knowledge, and to your neighbors afterwards by helping their infirmities. Some such I hope this Nation is worthy of, and to such I shall remain a friend during life, ready to my poor power to help.

After the introduction comes a list of authors quoted, a catalogue of herbs according to their planetary disposition and finally the description of English herbs in alphabetical order on 144 pages. Culpeper's *English Physitian* is basically a catalogue of 'simples', i.e. it lists names of medicinal plants in alphabetical order. Each plant is described according to four headings: (1) description, (2) place, (3) time, (4) government and virtues.

With this he follows the established format as used by Dodoens, Gerard and Parkinson. The only difference is that instead of classifying the virtues according to the 'temperature' or 'nature' of Galen's codex, Culpeper uses his astrological system, often combined with notes such as 'hot in the third degree'.

The Galenic principle goes back to Aristotle's system of the four elements: Fire, Water, Earth and Air. On this Galen based the hypothesis which ascribes to the properties of herbs and medicines

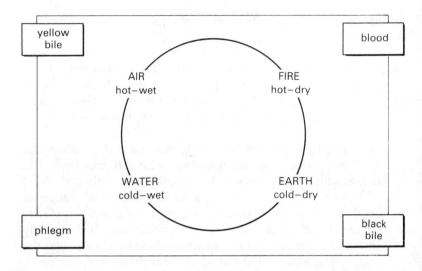

Figure 2.   The Artistotelean and Galenic Principles of Medicine

the four qualities or natures: 'Hot, cold, dryness and moisture.'
Health was defined as a maintenance of the right proportions of
these qualities in the body and disease an imbalance, e.g. having
too much heat. The therapeutic principle aimed at restoring the
proper balance by subtraction or addition of the right qualities.
Therefore, the virtue of plants were assessed from the point of view
of their heating and cooling property etc. Each quality existed in four
degrees. We thus find that a herb is hot or cold, moist or dry in the
first, second third or fourth degree.

In the astrological system a similar imbalance was supposed to
exist between the virtue of the stars with opposing pairs such as
Mars and Venus, Moon and Sun. The imbalance of disease was
treated by adding or subtracting, or by sympathy and antipathy,
between herbs belonging to one category or the other. Culpeper's
astrological system was therefore just as as arbitrary and unscientific
as the Aristotelian dogma. He says: 'Wormwood is an Herb of
Mars.' In the Galenic system according to Gerard it is 'hot and dry'.

At the end of the book follow 'Directions' or instructions about:
'gathering, drying and keeping simples and their juyces' plus
a pharmaceutical section devoted to 'Making and keeping compounds', and two pages about astrological concepts. By finally

adding 'An alphabetical catalogue of the diseases specified in this treatise, together with the page where to find it in the "English Physitian",' the *Herbal* became a complete guide of medicine and handy *vademecum* of therapeutics. No wonder it found its way into many households not only in England but also in all English-speaking countries of the New World and some colonies.

The publication was the labour of many years and represented Culpeper's most original ideas. Many herbals both large and small had appeared before and after Culpeper but none ever received as much popular acclaim as the *The English Physitian*. What was the reason for this?

As a declaration of purpose Culpeper starts by saying: 'In writing this work, first to satisfie myself I drew out all the virtues of vulgar herbs, plants and trees & cut of the best and approved authors I had or could get, and having done so, I set myself to study the reasons of them.'

A special feature of the *Herbal* was Culpeper's intention to explain the virtues of his medicines and to deduce their action from astrological concepts as already presented in his treatise *Semeiotica Uranica*, or 'Astrological Judgment of diseases'.[3] This was a novelty and Culpeper himself points out that similar messages were not available in the great leading herbals by Gerard and Parkinson.

Culpeper's new book was not intended to be a herbal in the conventional sense, which was to praise the virtues and beauties of plants, like Parkinson's the *'Paradise in sole'* or Gerard's *Herball, or general Historie of Plantes*; no, as apparent from the title it was supposed to be *the* English medicine book.

Culpeper's *English Physitian* sold like hot cakes. A mystery with Culpeper's book is why the humble little text became such an immediate and long-lasting success. The reasons were many: the book and its contents were selling arguments in itself and obviously it filled a demand at the right time. Health care in England for the vast majority of people was extremely poor. Not even in London were enough physicians available; and conventional medicines compounded according to the official pharmacopoeia and sold by the apothecaries were out of reach and far too expensive. The price of the book was right (three pence only), the text straightforward, easy to understand even for ordinary people, and the only requirement was the ability to read plain English.

The book sold well due to pre-publication publicity: it was written by Nicholas Culpeper, the astrologer, notorius for his courage to challenge the Physicians of London and author of many well-known tracts, almanacs and books. Then there was the special air about him; he had a reputation of being endowed with supernatural powers, and probably offered the *ultimate mystery* of the secrets of healing.

The first edition was a small folio which in the same year was followed by a pirate edition in *duodecimo*, half the size of the original, printed by a rival publisher, W. Bentley of London. Although Culpeper, like everybody else in the book trade, had to struggle with non existing copyright, the faked little handy pocket-book certainly helped enormously to make Culpeper's work popular and to increase its fame.

Culpeper was intensely personal in all of his descriptions, which sometimes struck a satirical note: 'Having gathered your herb, bruise it well in a stone mortar with a wooden pestle, than having put it into a canvas bag (the herb I mean not the mortar for that will yield but little juice).'

We can read between the lines and perceive a chuckle when Culpeper praises the 'retentive faculties' of medlar: 'The fruit stays fluxes and sure a better medicine he hardly hath to strengthen the retentive faculty; therefore it stays womens longings, the good old man cannot endure womens minds should run a gadding.'

Culpeper is of the opinion that God in his mercy makes medicines affordable and easily available to everyone. He writes about mistletoe which grows on different trees:

> Why that should have most vertues that grows upon oaks I know not, unless because 'tis rarest, and hardest to come by, and our Colledges opinion is in this contrary to the Scripture which saith, Gods tender mercies are over all his works, and easily available.
>
> Bees are industrious, and go abroad to gather honey from each plant and flower; but drones lie at home and eat up what the bees have taken pains for: just so do the College of Physicians lie at home and domineer, and suck out the sweetness of other men's labours and studies, themselves being as ignorant in knowledge of herbs as a child of four years old, as I can make appear to any rational man by their last dispensatory.

In *The English Physitian* we can trace an interesting innovation: the introduction of the Paracelsian concept of *similia similibus curantur* or 'similarities cure' instead of opposites, the Galenic principle. This principle is exemplified when Culpeper writes about 'Nettles': 'These are so well known that they need no description at all, they may be found by the feeling in the darkest night. They are good against itching, aches and gout.' This concept was later to become the tenet of homeopathy.

The *English Physitian* or the *Herbal* is by far Culpeper's most popular work, reprinted until our days (1983). Already in the 1813 edition by E. Sibly it says: 'This work has always been in great celebrity and request and has been many hundred times reprinted not only in England and Scotland but also in America.'[4]

Culpeper's *English Physitian* was later subject to a metamorphosis. A hundred and fifty years on, when the achievements of medicine-making had superseded old herbals, it became a publication on the fringe of medicine, the book it is today: an illustrated herbal, or colourful display of healing plants and manual of 'alternative' medicine.

In the eighteenth century the role of Culpeper's *Herbal* became a guide for household medicine; it was mainly read by women. One example is that of Charlotte Clark in 1755:

> She was taught French as soon as she could speak, she was never taught the use of needle work at all. She was sent to the country house of Dr. Hales, the physician, that in his family she might learn how to be a housewife, but it was now too late, she did not even learn how to provide an elegant table. At this place she got a smattering of physic. She was soon attended by many patients and with the assistance of Salmon and Culpepper, she recommended some remedy for every disease.[5]

It is worth considering what kind of herbals existed before the time of Culpeper: *The Herball* by John Gerard with 2146 woodcut illustrations appeared in print in 1597. It was the all-time favourite British herbal, which showed the author on the front page holding a novelty: the flowering potato plant. Gerard (1545–1612) was a barber surgeon with a passion for horticulture. He became herbalist to the King and had a celebrated garden in Holborn, where he grew more than a thousand plants, among them the potato which then was a rarity. He also superintended the gardens of Lord Burleigh in the Strand and at Theobalds. The 1636 edition 'General Historie of Plantes, very much enlarged and amended' was edited by the apothecary Thomas Johnson.

From Culpeper's publications it is evident that he was influenced by both Gerard and particularly Johnson, assistant of the Society of Apothecaries who organised the botanical expeditions in which Culpeper participated as an apprentice.

The *Paradisi in sole* (1629) and *Theatrum botanicum* (1640) by John Parkinson were the other sources for Culpeper's own herbal. Both of these were profusely illustrated with beautiful woodcuts and gave a desription of plants and flowers and advice about of their uses and virtues. John Parkinson (1567–1650) was apothecary to King James I and herbalist to Charles I. His house and garden were in Long Acre, near what is now Covent Garden. As we have seen, Parkinson had contributed to the original text of the *Pharmacopoeia Londinensis* of 1618.

Astrology was a serious matter to Culpeper and nothing less than divine revelation. Culpeper also recognised God's guidance in other aspects of his medical system. An important concept was the belief that God, the omnipotent Creator of health and disease, in his infinite mercy had also given mankind the proper remedy by the creation of medicinal plants according to the principle: there is a specific cure for every disease. Since people and diseases vary in different parts of the world, God accordingly had created a variety of herbs to fit the special needs in each country. This concept goes back to the Roman naturalist Plini and in England to Timothy Bright, the Elisabethan physician, better remembered as the inventor of modern shorthand.[6] On the Continent it was pursued by Paracelsus who introduced the concept of specifics.

During Culpeper's time the Doctrine of Signatures was widely accepted by all herbalists like Gerard, Johnson, Parkinson and Coles. Eyebright and chamomille were advocated as medicinal herbs for diseases of the eyes because their flowers looked like eyes. The concept that likeness of plants to certain organs was a key to therapy was called the 'Doctrine of Signatures'.

The belief that medicinal virtues of plants were signified by their appearance was thought to be an expression of the Creator's kindness to mankind. If he was all powerful and loving, why shouldn't he have labelled the plants for the information of his suffering man? It is actually written in the Bible:

The Lord hath created medicines out of the earth; and he that is wise will not abhor them. Was not the water made sweet with wood, that the virtue thereof might be known? And he has given men skill, that he might be honoured in his marvellous works. With such does he heal men and taketh away their pains. Of such doth the apothecary make a confection; and of his works there is no end; and from him is peace over all the earth.

Culpeper subscribed to this idea. He writes: 'Liverwort (with leaves resembling the liver) is a singular good herb for all the diseases of the liver. – Maidenhair this has very fine pale green stalks almost as fine as hair. Effectual in all diseases of the head and falling ot the recovering of hair.'

It may come as a surprise to find the foreign herb tobacco mentioned in Culpeper's herbal, but that is actually the case, although in the disguise of 'English Tobacco'. Culpeper, however, is of the opinion that exotic plants, once transferred to England and able to grow, change their virtues according to climate and soil and become appropriate to native inhabitants and their diseases.

Home-grown tobacco had seriously curtailed tax revenues of imported leaves. Therefore Parliament in 1651 passed an act prohibiting the planting of tobacco in England.[7] Culpeper wrote: 'It came from some parts of Brassilie and is more familier to our country than any of the other sorts. Nothing so large as the other Indian kinds.' Culpeper recommends it among other ailments: 'To be available to expectorate tough flegm from the stomach, chest and lungs. The seeds hereof is very effectual to help the toothache and the juice to kill lice in childrens heads.'

Vine is something that Culpeper extolls for certain purposes: 'The leaves of English vine (I do not intend to send you to the Canaries for a medicine) being boyled make a good lotion for sore mouths. The droppings of the vine when 'tis cut in spring, which country people calls tears, being boyled into a syrup with sugar and taken inwardly, is excellent to stay womens longings after everything they see, which is a disease many women and children are subject too.'

The Doctrine of Signatures was also framed to appeal to patriotism. Gerard in 1597 wrote:

Goldenrod is extolled above all other herbs for stopping of blood in sanguinolent ulcers and bleeding wounds; and has in times past been had in great estimation and regard and in these days: for I have known the dry herb which came from beyond the sea sold in Bucklersbury in London for half a crown an ounce. But since it was found in Hampstead wood, even as it were at our towns end, no man will give half a crown for an hundred weight of it: which plainly setteth forth our inconstancie and sudden unstabilitie, esteeming no longer of any thing, how pretious soever it be, than whilest it is strange and rare. This verifieth our English proverb, far fetcht and dear bought is best for ladies.

Yet it may be more truly said of phantastical physitians, who when they have found an approved medicine and perfect remedy neer home against any disese; yet not content therewith, they will seek for a new further off, and by that meanes many times hurt more than they help.[8]

Some, however, not only accepted the benevolent divine principle of signatures, but also believed that the devil could be involved and play his tricks to deceive men by making poisonous or useless herbs very similar to good ones.

Since his days in Isfield and during his apprenticeship as apothecary Culpeper had gained experience with herbs and learned from contemporary herbals such as Turner's, Gerard's and Parkinson's. A feature typical of all medical texts of the 16th and 17th centuries were the large number of quotations of reputable authorities like Galen and Dioscorides. Culpeper's *Herbal* mentions no less than 27 medical writers. The most frequently quoted authors besides Galen were Dioscorides and Pliny, those classical writers about *materia medica* whose works had served as a source of information to generations of Greek, Roman, Arabic and later north European physicians. The habit of citation was a common practice. Whenever possible, Dioscorides' and Pliny's accounts of therapeutic uses of herbal medicines would be supplemented by reference to some ancient Greek or Arabic physician. But a willingness to turn back to the ancients did not prevent Culpeper from criticizing the physicians and their dogma. This was new.

Culpeper was well aware of the misconceptions of the orthodox teachings of the physicians and their often dangerous therapeutic efforts. He said:

According to Hippocrates we have to consider three entities: the disease, the patient and the physician. The physician and the disease are mutual opponents and strive to fight a battle. Now the patient is subject and party in whom the battle between the two forces are fought. The physician should attack the disease and strengthen the patient in his own battle against the disease, but what do our learned physicians do in this battle? They weaken and harm the poor patient with their acrimonious and costly weapons. The prime aim really should be to strengthen the forces of natural defence by diet, healthy air and the God given elixirs of herbs!

No doubt, he had learned a great deal from his translation of the *London Pharmacopoeia*, not the least about the absurdities of polypharmacy (the mixing of many ingredients). While writing his *Herbal* he must actually have worked simultaneuosly on the second edition of the *Pharmacopoeia*, which becomes evident when comparing details of the two: In the *Pharmacopoeia* Culpeper adds comments about the virtues of Dwarf-Elder: 'The roots are as gallant a purge for the dropsie as any is under the sun, which was often proved by the never dying Dr. Butler of Cambridge, as myself have in a manuscript of his.'[9]

In the *Herbal* it says: 'Also Dr. Butler in a manuscript of his commends Dwarf Elder to the skye for dropsies.' This personal comment was included in both publications.

In another place in the *Pharmacopoeia* he wrote: 'The male (Fern) is that we in Sussex call Brakes'; and in the *Herbal*: 'The female fern is the plant which is in Sussex called Brakes.' Obviously a slight difference of opinion here, or a mistake?

When we today talk about Culpeper's *Herbal*, most of us think of a profusely illustrated coffee-table picture book with beautiful hand coloured engravings of herbs, flowers and shrubs. Illustrations of flowers was one of the charming features of late 18th and early 19th century editions, which could lead us to believe that this was one of the main reasons for their immense popularity. It may therefore come as a surprise to realise that the original first editions did not include a single picture of herbs! Obviously, therefore, the written content itself was immensely attractive and important to our forefathers.

It was not the ambition of Culpeper to produce an illus-trated herbal. Wood-cuts were excluded for many reasons: plant iconography was expensive and difficult to produce. We know this from the famous and expensive herbals of Gerard and Parkinson, both of whom obtained woodblocks from continental sources.[10] Since it was Culpeper's ambition to make his text available to all common people at a reasonable price, woodcuts had to be excluded. Moreover, Culpeper addressed readers who were still very much in touch with nature, knew their plants and needed no fancy pictures. He limited his botanical descriptions to a bare minimum and even excluded them altogether when he thought them not necessary. Time and again he omitted describing the herb: 'Plantane. This groweth so familiarly in meadows and fields, and by pathways, and is so well known that it needeth no description.'

And about Bur-Dock: 'it is so well known even to little boys who pull off the burs throw and stick upon one another, that I shall spare to write any description of it.'

Culpeper was always in a hurry; he was not friend of long-winded discussions. He said: 'I love brevity'.[11] He wanted to accomplish a lot in a short time: 'I shall not trouble you to make any repetition thereof, lest my book grow too big, but rather refer onto costmary with satisfaction, the vertues being the same.'

A lack of illustrations also characterised the most famous herbals by Theophrastus (3000 BC), Dioscorides (50 AD) and Plinius (60 AD) of the Greaco-Roman period. An illustrated edition of Dioscorides' *De materia medica* appeared in Constantinople in about 512 AD; the work of Theophrastus and Plinius never appeared with illustrations.[12]

Lack of illustrations in these early works cannot only be due to the fact that it would have been more difficult to reproduce pictures. The impact of the written word of these authors was sufficient to influence medicine for more than 1500 years! The 16th-century herbalist Brunschwig frankly stated: 'The figures are nothing more than a feast for the eyes, and for the information of those who cannot read or write.'

The only illustration in Culpeper's *Herbal* was a portrait of the author in a dark robe with long hair and a moustache. When we to-day look at this picture we might wonder if Culpeper really was a Puritan, or as they were called politically 'Roundheads' because of their short hair. The designation 'Roundheads' had already started during early Stuart times when, partly in reaction to the fashion at the court, short hair was adopted as a party badge. Later some ministers maintained that short hair was more scriptural. But only a few fanatics measured a man's faith and political opinion by the length of his hair.

Culpeper's *Herbal* covered cures for all known diseases from top to bottom. Here is just one example: 'The juyce of liquoris is effectual in all the diseases of the breast and lungs. The juyce dissolved in rose water with some gum tragacanth, is a fine licking medicine for hoarceness, weesings etc.'

We already know that he had a special interest in the diseases of women and their problems related to gestation and delivery. He certainly also was much engaged in pediatric medicine and for some reason he devoted an extra interest to diseases of the eye. We know this because he presents us with a long list of ophthalmic medicines (there are 44 entries about eye-diseases in the *Herbal*). He also tells us that he participated in the dissection of the eye of a sheep and a cat.[11] 'Distilled water of eyebright dropped into the eye or taken inwardly is worth a pair of spectacles. And if this herb were but as much used as it is neglected, it would half spoil the spectacle-makers trade.'[13]

An interesting quarrel between rival herbalists was that of William Coles and Nicholas Culpeper. Coles was an avid herbaliser and is known for his little book: *The Art of Simpling, an introduction to the knowledge and gathering of plants*. It appeared for the first time in 1656 and was reprinted the following year. Coles was a proponent of the Doctrine of Signatures just as Culpeper, but he disliked astrology. To Coles, Culpeper's astrological beliefs were sheer nonsense and he clearly expressed this in his book.

Coles' publication did not receive the wide acclaim of his rival and he therefore dedicated the second edition to the famous Elias Ashmole, an influential person and royalist, a friend of Lilly's and a proponent of astrology and alchemy. In the second edition he omitted the offending passages which critized astrology.[14]

Agnes Arber, who wrote the standard text about *Herbals, their origin and evolution* had, like many others, a preconveived opinion about Culpeper and the most popular herbal in the English language. She obviously disliked him because of his astrological comments, thereby 'throwing out the baby with the bathwater'. She does not like the 'bathwater', astrology, and likewise disregards the 'baby' – Culpeper's description of plants (which must have had immense importance for the dissimination of botanical knowledge among ordinary people in Britain). But Arber obviously did not take time to study Culpeper's writing properly since she mixes up the 'Physical Directory' (translation of the *London Pharmacopoeia*) with the *English Physitian* (Culpeper's *Herbal*).[15] A better judgment of the herbal is given by Rex Jones in his well balanced and extensively researched study: *Genealogy of a Classic: The English Physitian of Nicholas Culpeper.*[6]

The reaction to Culpeper's book was so overwhelming that two more editions were produced by other printers during the first year, and in 1653 another two editions were printed by Peter Cole.

Later re-issues of the 18th and 19th century abounded with hand-coloured plates. These editions were also very much changed in their contents, many mostly emphasizing so-called occult properties of herbs in a way which was not intended by Culpeper himself. One 1824 edition also added a gardening section: *The British Florist.* Particularly, the editions of Sibly (1798) and Gordon (1802) contain the description of a large number of plants not native to England, a fact that Culpeper would not have liked at all. In addition these books were intended to cover encyclopaedic knowledge in all fields of medicine, a 'know-it-all' and 'do-it-yourself' household treasure of medical knowledge.[4,16]

Culpeper's *Herbal* remained popular in the English-speaking countries all over the world for many years and even centuries later. It has been reprinted in different versions until this century, the latest edition appearing in 1983.

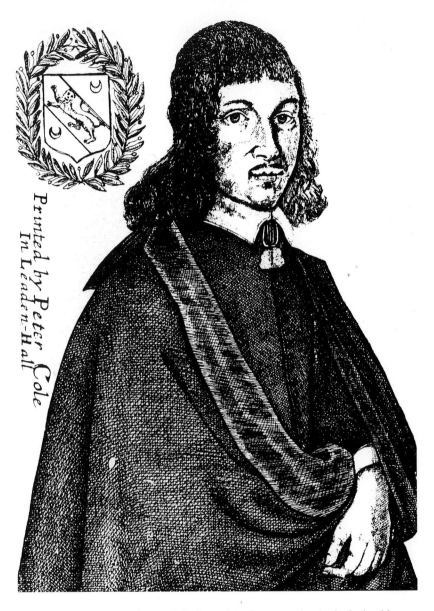

Printed by Peter Cole
In Leaden-Hall

1. Nicholas Culpeper (1616–54). One of the few portraits made during his life-time.

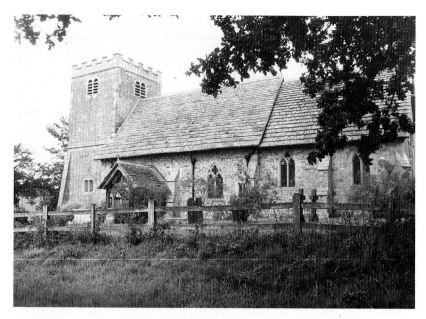

2. St Margaret's parish church of Ockley, Surrey. Here Culpeper's father was a vicar.

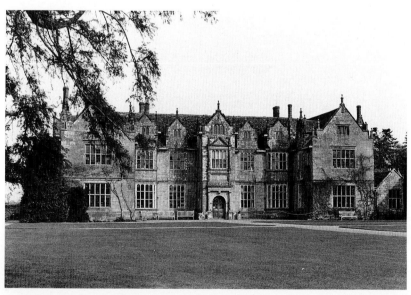

3. Wakehurst Place, Sussex. Manor house of the Wakehurst branch of the family to which Nicholas Culpeper belonged. It is surrounded by a beautiful park and now belongs to Royal Kew Gardens.

4. (right) St Margaret's parish church of Isfield, Sussex. Here young Nicholas sang as a chorister and spent many hours sitting in the pew listening to the sermons of his grandfather, the vicar William Attersoll.

5. (below) Old Vicarage of Isfield, Sussex. The only house still standing in which Nicholas Culpeper lived with his mother and grandfather.

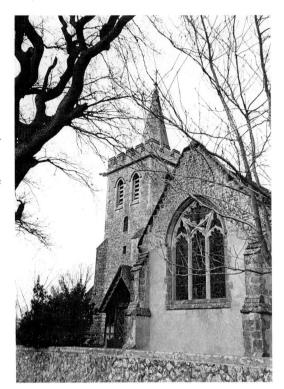

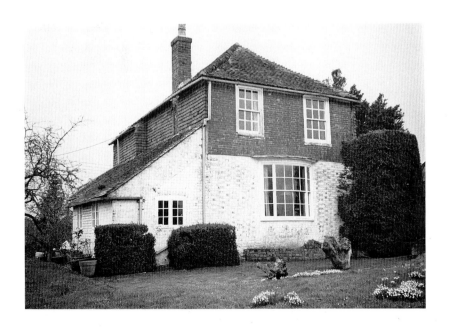

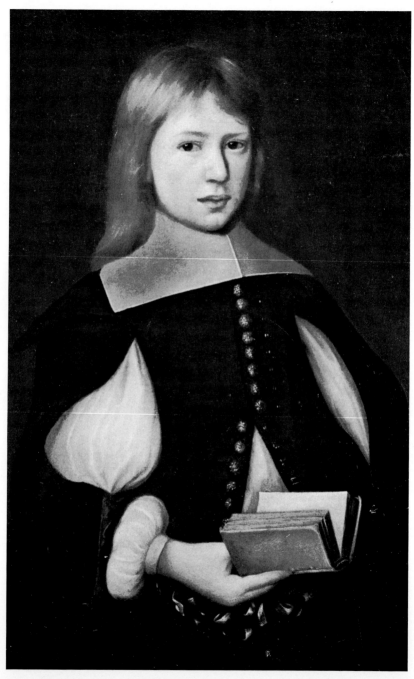

6. A Puritan schoolboy. This is how young Nicholas looked when he was a schoolboy at Lewes Grammar School.

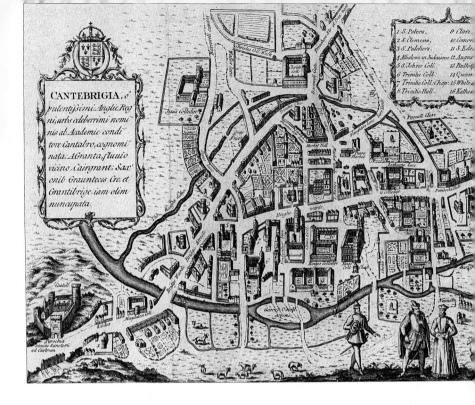

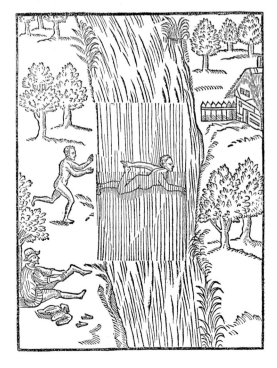

7. (above) Map of
    Cambridge with
    Colleges. A 17th-
    century print of the
    University town with an
    unusual projection:
    north is to the left.

8. (right) 'The art of
    swimming in Cambridge
    according to Digby.'
    Swimming was a
    forbidden but popular
    sport among college
    students.

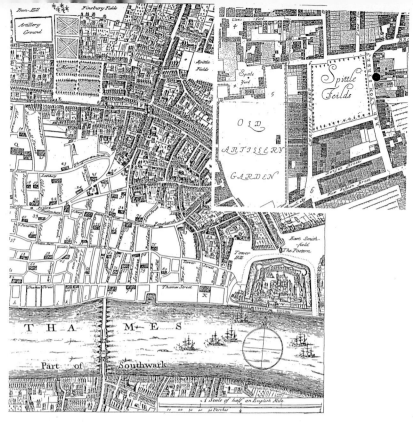

9. Map of North East London. It shows the location of Culpeper's house outside the City walls near Moorfields, not far from Shoreditch.

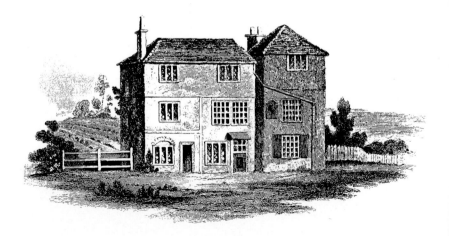

RED LION HOUSE, SPITALFIELDS.

IN WHICH CULPEPER LIVED, STUDIED AND DIED.

10. Culpeper's house in Spitalfields, London. It shows two houses built by Culpeper and a herb garden behind it.

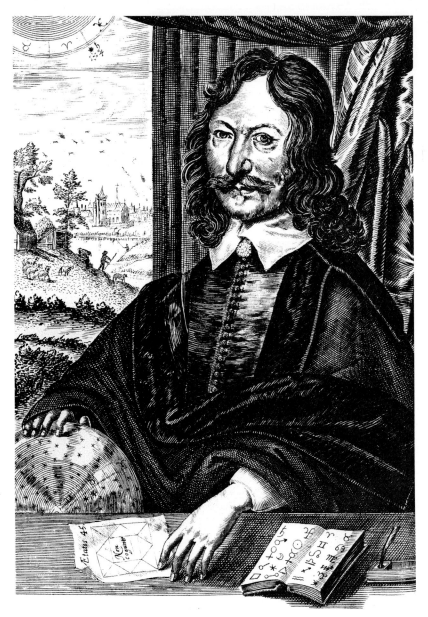

11.   William Lilly (1604–72). The famous astrologer and teacher of Culpeper.

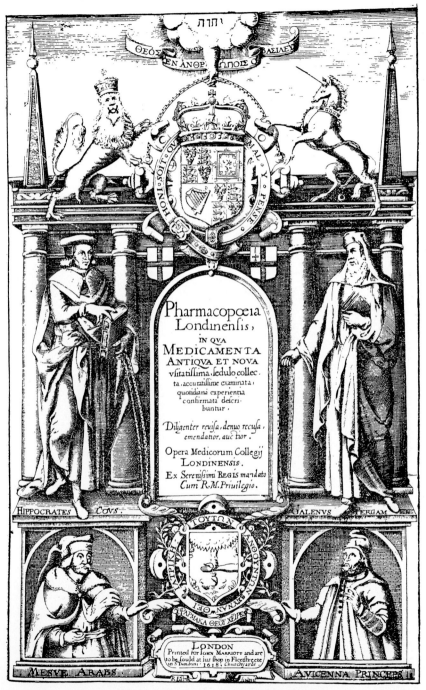

12. Title page of the Latin text of the *London Dispensatory* (1618). A translation of this text was Culpeper's first work.

A
𝒫 H Y S I C A L L
DIRECTORY

O R

A translation of the LONDON

DISPENSATORY

Made by the Colledge of Phyſicians in London.

*Being that book by which all Apothicaries are ſtrictly com-
manded to make all their Phyſick with many hundred additions which the reader may find in every page marked with
this letter* A.

*Alſo there is added the uſe of all the ſimples beginning at the
firſt page and ending at the* 78 *page.*

By 𝒩ich. Culpeper Gent.

Perſius.   *Diſce, ſed ira cadat naſo, rugoſaque ſanna.*
Cicere.   *Non nobis ſolum nati ſumus ſed etiam patrii.*

LONDON,

Printed for *Peter Cole* and are to be ſold at his Shop
at the ſign of the *Printing-preſſe* near to the
Royall Exchange 1649.

---

13.   *A Physicall Directory*, Culpeper's English translation of the *London
Dispensatory*, London, 1649.

THE
Englifh Phyfitian:
OR
An Aftrologo-Phyfical Difcourfe of the Vulgar
Herbs of this Nation.

*Being a Compleat Method of Phyfick, whereby a man
may preferve his Body in Health; or cure himfelf, being
fick, for three pence charge, with fuch things only
as grow in* England, *they being moft fit
for Englifh Bodies.*

Herein is alfo fhewed,

1. The way of making Plaifters, Oyntments, Oyls, Pultif-
fes, Syrups, Decoctions, Julips, or Waters, of all forts of
Phyfical Herbs, That you may have them readie for your
ufe at all times of the yeer.
2. What Planet governeth every Herb or Tree (ufed in
Phyfick) that groweth in *England.*
3. The Time of gathering all Herbs, both Vulgarly, and
Aftrologically.
4. The Way of drying and keeping the Herbs all the yeer.
5. The Way of keeping their Juyces ready for ufe at all
times.
6. The Way of making and keeping all kind of ufeful
Compounds made of Herbs.
7. The way of mixing Medicines according to *Caufe* and
and *Mixture* of the *Difeafe,* and *Part* of the Body *Afflicted.*

By *Nich. Culpeper,* Gent. Student in *Phyfick*
and *Aftrologie.*

LONDON:
Printed by *Peter Cole,* at the fign of the Printing-Prefs in
Cornhil, near the Royal Exchange. 1652.

14. *The English Physitian* (1652). Title page of the first edition of Culpeper's
famous herbal.

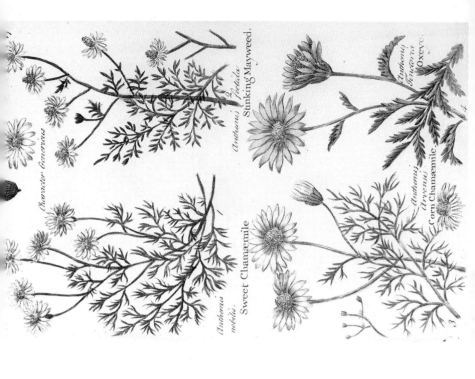

Chamæmelum Canariense

Anthemis nobilis
Sweet Chamæmile

Anthemis foetida.
Stinking Mayweed.

Anthemis Arvensis. Oxeye.

Anthemis arvensis
Corn Chamæmile

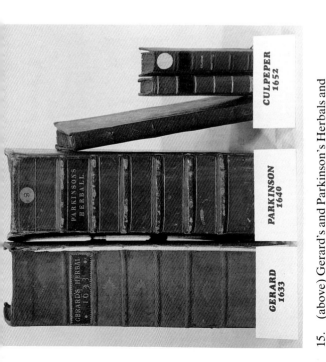

GERARD
1633

PARKINSON
1640

CULPEPER
1652

15. (above) Gerard's and Parkinson's Herbals and
     Culpeper's 1652 books. The juxtaposition shows the
     difference in size of the big and expensive publications
     and the successful popular books of Nicholas Culpeper.

16. (right) Illustrations from a 19th-century edition of
     Culpeper's *Herbal*. Illustrated editions of Culpeper's
     herbal first appeared in 1787.

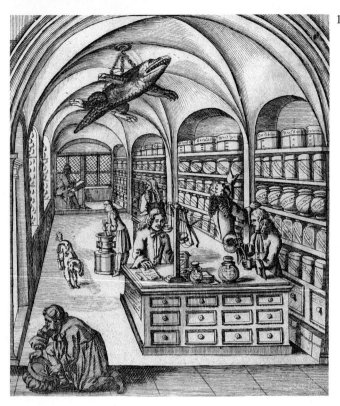

17. A 17th-century Pharmacy.

The Form the Child lies in, in the Womb, according to the Opinion of *Spigelius.*

This Table shews the Infant naked and disrobed of all its Tunicles, both Proper and Common.

18. Illustration from the *English Midwife* (enlarged), London, 1682.

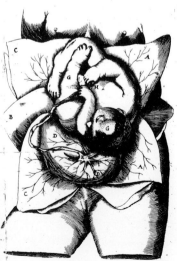

AA The portions of the Chorion *dissected and removed from their proper place.*

B *A portion of the Amnios.*

CC *The Membrane of the Womb dissected*

DD *The Placenta being a certain fleshy substance indued with very many Vessels, by which the Infant receives its Nourishment.*

E *The Varication of the Vessels which make up the Navel-string.*

FF *The Navel-string, by which, the Umbilicar Vessels are carried from the Placenta to the Navel.*

GG *The Infant as it lieth perfect in the Womb, neer the time of Travel.*

H *The Insertion of the Umbilicar Vessels into the Navel of the Infant.*

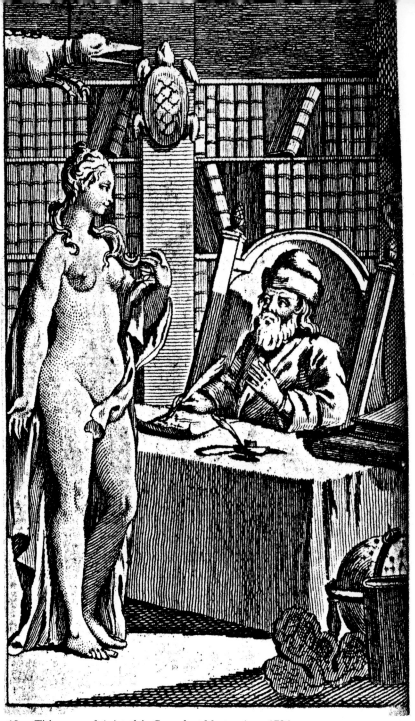

19.   Title page of *Aristotle's Compleat Masterpiece*, 1724.

20. Map of Virginia of 1651. It shows the parts of Virginia which Nicholas Culpeper's relatives owned, and depicts and praises the explorer Sir Francis Drake who 'discovered the happy shores . . . to the exeeding benefit of Great Brittain, and so to all true English'.

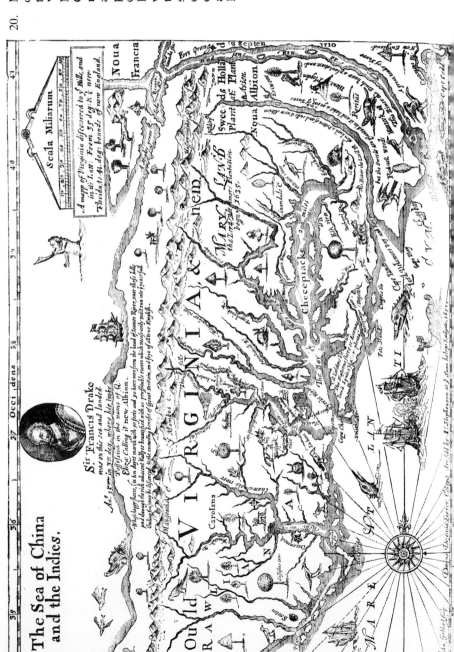

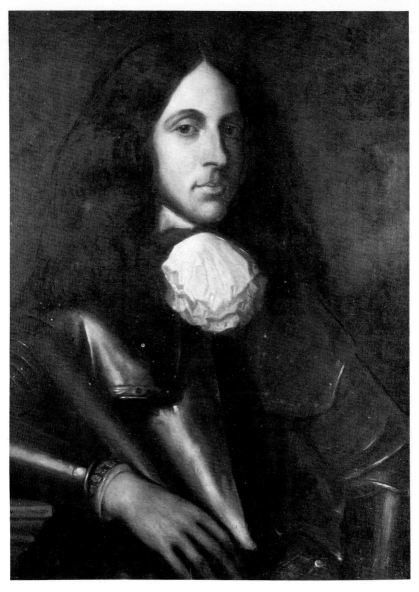

21. Thomas, Second Lord Culpeper of Virginia, an important relative of Nicholas Culpeper in the New World.

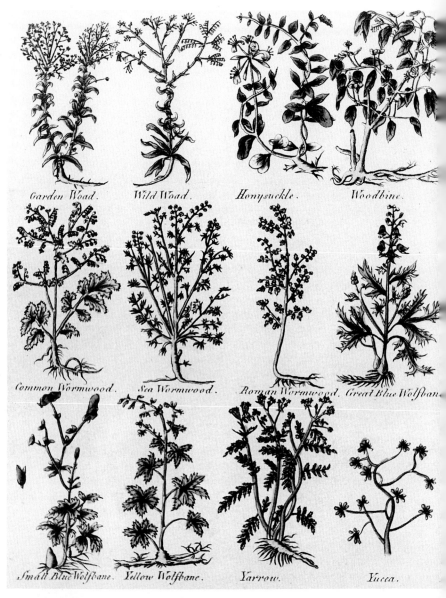

Garden Woad.   Wild Woad.   Honysuckle.   Woodbine.

Common Wormwood.   Sea Wormwood.   Roman Wormwood.   Great Blue Wolfban.

Small Blue Wolfbane.   Yellow Wolfbane.   Yarrow.   Yucca.

22.   Illustration of plants from Culpeper's *Herbal*, c. 1810.

11
Witchcraft & Starcraft

Go, and catch a falling star,
get with child a mandrake root,
tell me, where all past years are,
or who cleft the devil's foot.

John Donne, 1571–1631

The most flagrant expression of superstition in the seventeenth century was not astrology but the belief in witches and witchcraft. None of these absurd tendencies can be traced in Culpeper's work. The belief in witchcraft, however, was officially acknowledged by both King James I and Charles I.

On December 17, 1642, Culpeper himself was tried for witchcraft, an offence which could have resulted in a death-sentence. What was the charge? He was accused of 'having bewitched the widow Sarah Lynge, who languished until January 12 following'. He was found 'not guilty' and acquitted.[1] A mystery remains how such a charge could have been brought. The most likely explanation seems to be that he was accused by jealous physicians, who objected to his practice.

King James I, sometimes called 'the wisest fool in Christendom', firmly believed in witchcraft. Not to believe in witchcraft was impious in his opinion as not to believe in God. He felt deeply in the matter and set superstition going in England. He had grown up in Scotland in the midst of witch alarms. He believed that his own life had been influenced by witches. Before ascending the English throne he published his *Daemonologie*, a book on witchcraft. It is therefore not surprising that he introduced new strict legislation against witches. Before the new bill was passed it had been scrutinised by a large committee of experts including six earls and twelve bishops.

All witches except children should suffer death as a felon, i.e. any one who 'shall use, practise or exercise any invocation or conjuration of any evill and wicked spirit, or shall consult, convenant with, entertaine, employe, feede ot rewarde any evill and wicked spirit to or for any intent or purpose . . . For the first offence suffer one year's imprisonment with four appearances in the pillory, and for the second offence, death if he or she hurte or destroy any person in his or her bodie . . . ' (The latter citation was probably applied to Culpeper when he was accused of witchcraft).

In the royal directions for trying witches a water-immersion test was recommended: the accused was bound crosswise hand and foot with a rope around his/her waist. If the accused sank, she was innocent but if she floated she was guilty because the pure water of baptism had rejected her. The law was enforced with vigour and during the first fifteen years of James reign 50 people suffered the death penalty.

In his attitude towards superstition Charles I resembled his father in his later years. There were six executions from 1625 to the time Civil War broke out. The Lancashire witches of 1633 were the most notorious cases during this period and William Harvey supervised their examination together with two other physicians, five surgeons and ten midwives. Although the tests did not give positive evidence of witchcraft the accused were not released from prison because the King was reluctant to antagonise public sentiment by declaring them innocent, particularly since one woman had confessed her guilt. The Protectorate was less eventful but at the Restoration the practice of witchcraft again flared up and during this period Elias Ashmole and the Royal gardener John Tradescent were busy attending witch trials.[2] The last legal hanging of a witch in England took place in 1722; but even after 1736, when the laws against them were repealed, there were many who advocated their death.[3]

In astrology one of the guiding principles, as in science, is the tenet of cause and effect. This was also sought. Primitive man had learned that daily life and seasons characterised by light and darkness, heat and cold, were associated with the cycles of the sun, moon and stars. It was noticed that the sun ruled and vitalised the earth as evident from the seasonal changes of winter, spring and summer. Furthermore it could not be denied that the moon had a profound influence on tidal waters. People saw these effects of the sun and the moon; why, they argued, could not other planets induce similar things? It was natural, then, to suppose that the overruling power which determines the apparent changes of human life, is in the heavens, and that by proper observation one should be able to make predictions from the movement of the stars.

This led to a search for other celestial signs. If the appearance of a comet or eclipse was noted simultaneously with the death of a great man or the scorge of an epidemic this could be interpreted as cause and effect. Therefore it was the ambition of many star gazers and astronomers to record the occurrence of comets, new stars, eclipses, meteors and remarkable constellations of planets as well as plagues, deaths and wars. Thereafter they thought they could trace a causal relationship which might lead them to predict diseases and disasters.

To the astrologer a knowledge of the stars was not essential to explain physical laws (such as gravity) but valuable only as a means of foretelling future events and to help in the cure of diseases. Similarily the alchemist worked not with the view of discovering chemical properties of substances, but to produce gold and silver and of finding a panacea for the cure of diseases.

Astrology can be divided into two branches: natural and judicial. Astral influences on the weather, tides and plants belong to the first category and predictions and advice about personal and political matters concern the latter. Natural astrology deals with the existence and influence of rhythms. To say the moon and tides run in cycles of 28 days is to state a fact of natural astrology. Judicial astrology is concerned with prediction of future events. The meaning of the planets was interpreted from the point of their symbolic individual qualities such as hot or cold, dry or wet. In this way, each planet was held to signify or 'rule' different matters such as individuals, herbs, the weather etc. Astrological medicine mainly belongs to the judicial branch. A justification for this pseudo-science was, among other things, the view that rhythmical events like the menstrual cycle were under the influence of the moon just as the lunar influenced the mood ('lunatic'). Astrological physicians would diagnose the disease, predict its course, and prescribe for it on the basis of this prediction – often merely by casting a horoscope for a patient they had not even seen.[4] Lilly and Culpeper clearly practised judicial astrology.

Culpeper's own opinion about astrology was: 'The art which teachest the meaning of God towards men' and he supports his view by quoting Genesis 1: 15–18. 'God made the sun, moon and stars to rule over night and day . . . to be signs of things to come.'

The charts to describe judicial astrology were called figures, nativities or horoscopes. A nativity was based on the time and place of birth and the corresponding planetary constellation. Since many people did not know the exact time of their births to enable casting a nativity, predictions based on planetary position at the time and place of enquiry became more popular and were called 'horary' predictions. Astrology so penetrated the common and general attitude of belief that it has left innumerable metaphors in our language.

Astrology, the expression of man's impatient curiosity of the unknown and desire for rational explanation, emerged as an attempt of man to explain the vagaries of life and to obtain rules by which to live. The upswing of astrology during the time of the Civil War and the Commonwealth can be considered a natural consequence of the turmoil and unrest which affected all spheres of life. Astrologers played an important role in the struggle between Roundheads and Cavaliers to decide whether Parliament or King should rule the country; they were the psychological warfare experts of their time, fabricating predictions designed to keep up the morale on either side. In London, Lilly prophesied the success of Parliament and in Oxford, the headquarters of King Charles I, Royalist astrologers asserted the opposite.[5] People were confused, whom should they believe? The situation was like the turmoil in ancient Babylon with the inability of the Chaldean astrologers to tell the truth. This is aptly described by Isaiah: 'Thou art wearied in the multitude of thy counsels. Let now the astrologers, the star-gazers, the monthly prognosticators, stand up, and save thee from these things that shall come upon thee.'

As we have seen, astrology was highly political and could be used to predict anything: the overthrow of monarchy or the importance of maintaining hierarchy. Clearly two camps developed: one egalitarian which supported Parliament and the other anti-democratic and royalist. Culpeper belonged to the former and Elias Ashmole (1617–1692) was the epitome of the latter. Ashmole was a founding father of the Royal Society of London, interested in all kinds of natural sciences, magic and alchemy. Lilly was smart in that most of the time he bet on the winning horse. In the beginning he was clearly pro-Parliament and predicted their decisive victory in the Civil War at Naseby in 1645, but even at the Restoration he managed to carry on his work and Elias Ashmole became one of his greatest supporters at court. In the end Lilly was granted permission to practice medicine by the Archbishop of Canterbury, the only qualification for the job being his knowledge of astrology.

There was constant speculation about the immediate future and personal security. All signs of nature were eagerly anatomised as to whether they could be used to predict the coming of a new paradise on earth, a Fifth Moncharchy, or heralded disaster. English astrology reached unprecedented heights of popularity and influence. This can simply be inferred from the large production and consumption of astrological almanacs, books and pamphlets in the seventeenth century. One reason for the vast proliferation of all kinds of astrological literature was the nearly unlimited liberty of the press. Between 1641 to 1660 the strict censorship by the monarchy and church broke down and it became easier for eccentrics to get into print.[5]

This period of English history, as never before or after, was characterised by the underworld of occult medical literature. In an avalanche of books, tracts and alamanacs it is easy to discard everything as rubbish. Among the vast numbers of synopses, astrological judgements, animadversions, secrets etc. we may also discover such important works as Robert Burton's *The Anatomy of Melancholy* and Culpeper's *English Physitian,* one dealing with affections of the mind and the other with medicine.

While in the seventeenth century doubts about judicial astrology emerged it is fair to say that the influence of the stars on natural phenomena was still universally accepted. Judicial astrology, however, survived mostly because it was aided by superstition and fear of the future. John Evelyn believed in the influence of stars and admired the astrologer William Lilly. Samuel Pepys bought a book written in 1642 that predicted great events for 1666.

Judicial astrology has always been favoured by politicians and there were many court astrologers. Bernard Capp relates that the French court astrologer Morin was concealed in the royal bedroom to record the precise moment when the young Louis XIV and his bride consummated their marriage, in order to calculate the horoscope of the dauphin who would hopefully be conceived.[5] Belief in nativities and horoscopes was hard to kill, particularly if the astrologers, like Lilly, added the caveats *'astra non cogunt',* the stars do not compel, but they incline and *'homo sapiens dominabitur astris',* the wise man will rule his stars.

From our present vantage-point it is hard to believe that in the century of Bacon, Harvey, Boyle, Wren and Newton astrology flourished like never before. If we take a closer look we will discover that many respected mathematicians and astronomers were also astrologers. It is significant that most contemporary scientists looked upon astrology as applied astronomy. Even a sceptical Francis Bacon acknowledged that astronomy owed much to the study of planetary influence, as chemistry had its debts to the alchemists.

In order to fully appreciate the importance of natural astrology it is helpful to listen to what Francis Bacon had to say. In his treatise about winds Bacon believed that the study of planetary influences could be useful:

> Enquire sparingly concerning astrological considerations of winds, what meteors of several sorts do . . . these things are linked together . . . let all manners of prognostics of winds be carefully gathered together. In the prediction of the weather he said: 'As for astrology, it is so full of superstition, that scarce anything sound can be descivered in it. Notwithstanding, I would rather have it purified than altogether rejected.'[6]

Religion and astrology both belong to the sphere of the supernatural and therefore overlapped. It was not difficult to reconcile astrology and religion because from the Christian point of view the stars were created by the omnipotent God and could be regarded as his messengers to mankind: the shining planets being a looking glass to heaven, a link to the Creator. It was the task of the astrologer to interpret the celestial language, the harbinger of good news and admonitions.

Critics stigmatised astrology as superstition and as being opposed to free will and moral responsibility. But the famous astrologer William Lilly in 1647 succeeded to convince most critics with his textbook *Christian Astrology*, which became an immediate success. Lilly regarded astrology as a divine craft which gave him the gift of prophecy. It was Lilly who prophesied the 1655 Great Plague and the Fire of London of 1666.

One of the strangest examples of 17th-century quackery was Sir Kenelm Digby's weapon-salve, or powder of sympathy. This mysterious medicine was advocated for the treatment of wounds inflicted in combat and was applied not to the wound but (after it had been inflicted) to the weapon! It was of ancient but obscure origin. Digby, a man of prominence, ambassador to foreign countries and member of the Royal Society, popularised its use. Digby advocated that the preparation, which was mainly powdered vitriol, never be brought in contact with the wound. A bandage was to be taken from the wound, immersed in the powder and kept there till the wound healed.[7] It was probably just as well that the ointment was not applied to the wound because of its strange composition. This type of treatment may look very simple but there was one drawback: one could not always obtain the weapon for anointment. Sometimes the enemy disappeared with his sword or dagger. Digby's great contribution was that it was not necessary to have access to the weapon – a bloodstained bandage from the victim's wound was enough and could always be made available! There were of course many favourable testimonials about the weapon-powder from those who were fortunate enough to recover. Those who did not recover often died and were silent! Similar methods of treatment were also tried by applying sympathetic powder to the urine of patients with fevers.

Digby was an astrologer and alchemist. He also cast his own horoscope but did not have the courage to make it come true because he was alive when the predicted date of his demise occurred, unlike Robert Burton, the author of *The Anatomy of Melancholy*, who died as predicted in 1640. Legend has it that the author killed himself on the day predicted by his horoscope in order to verify his astrological belief.

It is significant to note that before the institution of the Royal Society (which was devoted to science) there was a Society of Astrologers of London. This association of 40 astrologers existed between 1647 to 1658 and Culpeper was an active member. When he attended their meetings he also must have had some arguments with his political opponents, the royalist astrologers.

In 1652 he commented: 'Dr Gell in his last sermon preached before the learned Society of Astrologers.' Here he delivered lectures on astrological medicine ('certain astrological lectures which I read'). Later in 1651 they were published in a book as '*Semeiotica Uranica*, or astrological judgment of diseases, what planet caused it and what planet cured it by sympathy and antipathy.'

Culpeper's astrological training goes back to an early age in Isfield through the influence of his grandfather and his books. Culpeper quotes the 1603 book of Sir Cristopher Heydon, *A defence of judiciall Astrology* which Attersoll must have had in his library. Later he was trained by William Lilly whom he reverently quotes:

> It was the opinion of Mr. Lilly in that masterpiece of his, 'Prophetical Merlin.' But he does not blindly follow his teacher:
> 'I hope Mr. Lilly will pardon me if I dissent a little from him: if he may freely write his own judgment, why may not I by the same rule'?[8]

The most controversial of Culpeper's book was his '*Catastrophe Magnatum*, or the fall of Monarchie, a caveat to Magistrates deduced from the eclipse of the sunne, March 29 1652 with a probable conjecture of the determination of the effects.' This treatise predicts the coming of a new age, a change of rule in England and hopeful predictions for the future.

He starts by explaining what an eclipse is: 'The prohibition of the light of the sun or moon from our eye.' He goes on to relate previous eclipses and their meaning and claims that there will be an eclipse of the moon on March 14, 1652 and of the sun on March 29, 1652.

In his busy practice he did not have the time to make all the calculations but employed:

> 'My special and loving friend Samuel Warre to calculate this eclipse for me by the tables of Bullialdus.'
> The message was: 'Violent storms and unusual, if not unheard of hail will be prejudice unto the earth, especially towards the later end of the summer 1652, 1653 and its well of 1654 escape.' . . . 'The fifth Monarchy is coming but he is not Scotchman nor English.'

Culpeper seemed to imply the coming of someone like King Gustavus Adolphus of Sweden, an idealialised champion for many, who on the Continent fought for protestantism. It also meant that he was not in favour of a noted Englishmen, Oliver Cromwell, who was to become Lord Protector in 1653, something Culpeper did not predict. 'Beware of pestilence 1653, get able physitians.' . . . 'In the year 1654 England begins to grow quiet and I am glad of that, she enjoys her desired liberty.' . . .

Culpeper was not as lucky as Lilly in his predictions but he was clever enough to add the following wise comment, as if anticipating his failure: 'A few years will show whether what I have written be true or false. – Imagine what I write be every word false, what harm will it do princes to prepare for the loss of a kingdom though it never come. Is it not the way to teach them humility?'

The publication created an upheaval, this time not from the royalists, but from Cromwell. Culpeper predicted the demise of all established governments and the coming of a new age under the divine guidance of Christ and his Saints.

> Black Monday occurred on March 29th 1652. It was the fearfullest ecclipse of the sun ever seen by mankind. It came on at about nine in the morning: a day of much obscurity, darker and darker. Ploughmen unyoked their teams, birds sorrowfully chirping took to roost, men in amazement to prayer. A day of much obscurity, stars came out. This event was much noised about by Lilly, Booker and other astrologers like Culpeper.[9]

An eclipse was something that not only interested learned men with their telescopes and astrologers, but deeply affected the mind of everybody since it was an expression of a celestial event for everybody to see. It is therefore not surprising that it was interpreted by almost everybody as a terrible presage of dire events. This, together with the political turmoil of the past ten years, must have given nourishment to Culpeper's astrological inclinations to continue making forcasts about the future, despite the fact that the eclipse in 1652 was not as anticipated. Almanacs with forecasts appeared for the years 1651, 1652 and 1653 in his name.

In 1653 a broadsheet appeared which expressed the general opinion of the time:

> What learned astrologers writeth this yeare.
> I purpose now unto you for to declare,
> especially Lilly a man of great learning,
> in famous astrology by your discerning.
> And likewise Culpeper, a man of great fame
> known all over England edem by this name.
> What they fortold you here shall find,
> strange and remarkable it is you will minde.
> Feavers and other diseases most strange
> about the city and country will range.

Culpeper was not alone in his prediction of the 1652 eclipse of the sun and its dire consequenses. Lilly also published a similar tract, but he predicted the fall of Parliament and condemned Fifth Monarchists. The solar eclipse actually happened but without dire consequences. This resulted in pamphlets entitled: '*Mercurius Phreneticus*' and '*Mercurius Democritus*' which ridiculed Culpeper and Lilly. 'Philastrogus Knavery' was another tract which tried to vindicate Culpeper and Lilly. The predicted revolutionary changes never happened but both Culpeper and Lilly were seized, accused of treason and briefly imprisoned. In the State Papers we read: 'The book published by Mr Culpeper referred to the Committee for examinations, who are to send for and examine him thereon, or any other person who have had any hand in its contriving, printing, or publishing, and secure them if they see cause.'

In the seventeenth century astrology was part of everyday life and not something only for horoscope charts and quack-medicine. It is quite revealing to read John Parkinson's 1629 *Flower Garden*. He is puzzled by the fact that some daisies, daffodils and anemones grow double flowers. He tries different ways of planting and nursing but cannot arrive at a rational explanation why he sometimes succeeds to get big double flowers and sometimes not. Therefore he concludes that it may have something to do with 'The change of the Moon, the constellations or conjunctions of Planets, or some Stars or celestial bodies'.[10]

But already in the 16th century voices could be heard against astrology. Jean Calvin wrote 'An admonition against astrology judiciall and other curiosities', but he made a small reservation: 'We must needes confesse that there is a certain convenience betwyxte the starres or planets and the dispocion of man's body.' The most rational critic of his time was William Fulke who even discredited the validity of astrology in medicine: 'sycknesse and healthe depende upon divers causes, but nothyng at al upon the course of the starres, for what way soever the starres runne their race, yf there be in the body abundance or defect, or from outward by corruption of the ayre infection it must nedes be sycke: and if none of these bee, though all the starres in heaven with all their oppositions and evil tokens shuld meete in the howse of sickness, yet the boddy should bee whole, and in good healthe.'[11]

We might think that medical starcraft should have been obsolete in a century of Enlightenment. Was the seventeenth century emerging from the Renaissance not the age of rationalism with men like Francis Bacon, William Harvey and Thomas Sydenham? Astrology was still so deeply rooted in the opinion of the time that it is difficult to find any medical treatises which show no traces of it. On the one hand the Galenists, who represented the conservative classical school, inherited a large amount of astrological doctrine along with their physiology of the four humors. On the other hand the chemical physicians who stemmed from Paracelsus and Van Helmont, and who were the most vigorous proponents of Baconian empiricism, were also entangled with the doctrine of signatures and sympathies which in origin were altogether astrological. Christopher Hill aptly states: 'we cannot separate the early history of science from the history of magic, cannot give prizes to good rationalists against bad magicians, astrologers, alchemists. Most men and women in the seventeenth-century Britain still lived in a world of magic, in which God and the devil intervened daily, a world of witches, fairies and charms'.[12]

Both Galenic and Paracelsian medicine contained elements of astrology. Only a minority looked upon astrology as a pseudo-science and condemmed the practice as being humbug. Therefore Culpeper was not in bad company when he declared that astrology is a 'part of natural philosophy which inquires after causes, properties, nature and effects of starres'.

The Aristotelian-Galenic principles and astrology so dominated the minds of everybody that even staunch naturalists such as Francis Bacon, Robert Boyle and William Harvey clearly exhibited the stamp of their time. In Bacon's words: 'The breaths in man's microcosmos do very well agree with the winds in the greater world. For they are engendered by humours, and alter with moisture as wind and rain doth.' Further in the same treatise about 'The Natural and Experimental History of the Forms of Hot Things', Bacon goes on to say: 'Drugs that are sharp and biting upon the palate, much more being taken inward are perceived to be hot . . . Some vegetables are hot and some are cold. Among vegetables there is not any plant that seems hot being touched but the inward feeling as that of the palate and stomach.'

From the gustatory perception of 'hot' and spicy he adds another dimension of heat when he says: 'The carcasses and dung have the potential kind of heat. For horse dung itself retains no heat unless it be laid close up, this also applies to green leaves. There is a kind of heat in putrified things such as flesh and cheese which putrified turn into maggots.'[13] This view is shared by 17th-century physicians who prescribed excrements, which are mentioned in the *London Pharmacopoeia*.

In analogy to the thermal effect of herbs which are not necessarily perceived by the skin he says: 'According to astronomers there are some stars hotter than others. And amongst the planets next to Sol, Mars is the hottest, then Jupiter and then Venus. Luna is cold and Saturn coldest of all. . . . Sol, and likewise the rest of the planets are thought to yield a greater heat when they are nearest to the greatest fixed starres, as when Sol is in Leo, than when it is in cancer. It is credible that the parts of heavens doe infuse the greater heat, though it be not perceptable to the feeling, the more they are adorned with stars, especially of the biggest kinde.'

Bacon tries to explain the difference of celestial heat by the effect of burning glass and the distance to objects as if the rays of the stars were magnified by adjacent planets. This means that Bacon clearly subscribes to the common opinion of the influence of stars by virtue of the heat they exert on the human body even if this is not directly felt on the skin. He further goes on to describe the physiology of heat: 'Living creatures have their heat increased in them by motion and exercise, by wine and high food, venery, burning feavers and pain.'[13]

Also Robert Boyle made concessions when he said 'I am not willing to deny . . . that there are any such things as coelestial influences, by which I mean powers whereby coelestial bodies may act upon sublunary ones, otherwise then by their light, or their heat'.[14]

When judging the life-work of Nicholas Culpeper we must take into consideration that he was a product of his time. His medicines often were innocent placebos and most of them certainly did not harm the patient. On the contrary they often did the patient good and instilled confidence. The astrological medicine of Culpeper should deserve a sympathetic hearing since even precise and proper boundaries of science and fiction were not clearcut even to venerated scientists. Isaac Newton devoted no less time to alchemy and religion than he did to physics and mathematics. Harvey, the epitome of scientific medical enquiry of his time, probably reflects the general opinion of his contemporaries. He talks about the use of horoscopes to predict the birth of boys or girls.[15] Therefore the vast corpus of ancient lore of astrology never disappeared, but was worn away by slow attrition and finally transformed to an empty shell of superstition.[12]

The main criticism of Culpeper today, which gave him the epithet of a quack forever, had to do with the fact that he dabbled in occultism and astrology. How could a serious doctor believe in such rubbish? There is a certain irony when one considers that the work of Culpeper was ridiculed because he practised astrology, but nobody mentions that even scientists like Kepler, Bacon, Harvey and Newton had astrological inclinations. We tend to be quick to judge, but we must realise that in this illuminated time of ours the impact of occultism, despite all scientific achievements, is immense. Horoscopes are a regular feature in modern magazines and newspapers and a very large number of people watch horoscopes on national television (in Britain); also, the sale of occult literature, such as, the teachings of Nostradamus, is significant!

In 1792 'The Conjuror's Magazine, or Magical and Physiognomical Mirror' published in the name of Peter the nativity of Culpeper which in most parts was copied from John Gadbury.[16] The interpretation given was:

> The sign ascending the horoscope is capricorn, a sign of brevity, and saturn, the lord of the ascendant, is in taurus, a sign of brevity also, the Moon in the sixth house, decreasing in light; all which are arguments of a middle stature, and somewhat of a spare, lean body, complexion darkish, or swarthy, hair dark brown, visage more long than round, eyes quick and piercing and the person of this nativity was exactly such; and he was also full of agility, very active and nimble, which I presume was occasioned by the moon's position in the house of mercury in sextile to mars and saturn in the house of venus, having south latitude.
>
> His temperature, according to astrologers, should be melancholy, choleric, as is plain by an earthy sign ascending, and saturn's position in an earthy sign also, and the moon being among martial fixed stars, and stars of the same nature in the ascendent are very strong testimonies of choler prevailing over this native; but the greatest testimony of choler predominating, I take to be the sun's reception with mars from violent signs, which seems to signify that choler should overpower the humour of melancholy, notwithstanding an earthy sign ascending. He was indeed of such temperature, that melancholy was an extraordinary enemy unto him, so great at some times, that wanting company he would seem

like a dead man; and at other times would his choler afflict him very strangely, even more than melancholy.

Mercury, the patron of ingenuity, is the most potent planet in the figure, and being in scorpio, the house of mars, and so near benevolent beams of venus, argued the native to be of an excellent wit, sharp fency, admirable conception, and of an active understanding. For proof of this let many worthy works extant be summoned to give in evidence . . . He was eloquent, a good orator, spoke both freely and fluently and if I should speak the truth he was very conceited (full of ideas), and full of jests as the square of mars to mercury denotes . . .

It is most true, that he was always subject to a consumption of the purse, notwithstanding the many ways he had to assist him. His patrimony was chiefly consumed at the university, he had a spirit so far above the vulgar that he contemned and scorned riches . . . Now mars, lord of the eleventh in square to four planets, denotes the native's friends, or at least such as pretend friendship unto him, to be hypocritical and deceitful.

Before discoveries in astronomy, science and anatomy killed traditional ideas of the Middle Ages a long process of awakening was necessary. The beginning was made in the fifteenth and sixteenth century with the spread of information through the invention of printing and international communication. An important step in this process was the translation of the Bible into English, which was largely the consequence of the Reformation in the mid sixteenth century, although there had been earlier attempts. The most notable was the English Bible of John Wycliffe, written in 1382–88. This, however, was banned and burned by the Church. Moreover, the impact was not great because the translation occurred before the invention of printing. The first official English Bible was the 'Great Bible' of 1539, based on William Tyndale's translation which was ordered to be used in churches and remained standard until the appearance of the famous 'Authorised Version' of King James in 1611.

With the availability of cheap Bibles it was no longer the privilege of the Church to interpret the teachings of God and to spread the Gospel among the people. Every man was his own preacher. It was Culpeper's ambition to do the same for health care and folk medicine and to obviate the need for physicians. Before the advent of hospital care and the technicalities of specialisation this was a realistic possibility.

The vernacular Bibles became an eye-opener to many, including the clergy. Catholics maintained that it was sinful to translate the holy text and clerics were not even expected to read God's word in Hebrew or Greek but the authorised version in Latin, the *Vulgata*. This was the Latin version of St Jerome, made in the fourth century and first printed by Gutenberg in 1450.

The physicians were of the same opinion as the clerics, that the official medical texts were the privilege of the learned and should not be translated into the vernacular. Culpeper compares himself to the translators of the Bible when he says: 'I confess many excellent books have of late been printed in our own mother tongue. In divinity they have given us a translation the Bible. The scripture is a mysterious piece, each word will teach you knowledge . . . I write for children and milk is fittest food for them.'[17]

Latin was the accepted *lingua franca* of the scientific and medical world. This had the advantage that texts written in Germany, Denmark or France could be read not only by scholars in these countries but also elsewhere all over the world. The situation resembles international scientific communication of today which is primarily based on English. In the 17th century men like Bacon, Boyle and Sydenham all published in Latin.

Medical books in Latin, however, did not help to improve health education in England. Problems of comprehension gave rise to misunderstanding and errors occurred with medical treatises and rules for prescription of drugs. This was the concern of Nicholas Culpeper who saw himself as educator of the common man. To him this was like a religious calling, like translating the Bible, to make medical texts available not only to a select elite but to everybody.

The time of the Civil War in England was not only a military confrontation between Parliament and the King. It was much more, it was also a social, religious and moral revolt. Christopher Hill characterises the situation as 'The world turned upside down'.[12] Accepted standards of society were questioned and many new movements emerged like the Levellers, Ranters Baptists and Quakers.

During the period of 1642 to 1660 censorship of the press practically disappeared or was liberalised and the public was flooded with cheap books, pamphlets, tracts and almanacs. In 1641 the Bohemian educator Comenius was invited by supporters of parliament to give advice for the reform of English education. Comenius made radical recommendations: he advocated general education for both boys and girls alike, using the vernacular and not Latin to improve the situation of the lower classes. Comenius and before him Francis Bacon, were optimists who believed that knowledge and skills could better mankind.[12]

Culpeper was deeply influenced by these radical ideas. Time and again in the introduction to his books he mentions the importance of learning and information of the common people, and castigates the suppression of knowledge:

> Unless a man have gotten a very large estate he is not able to bring up his son to understand Latin. A dozen years of expense of time will hardly do it as they have ordered matters, in which time, by whipping and cruel usage the brains of many are too stuped that they are unfit for study. People miserably hampered by a scholastical net that they cannot get out if they do see it. The righteous God look upon poor people and redeem them out of such Egyptian bondage.[18]

If we want to judge the importance of Culpeper from a contemporary historical perspective it is not the introduction of his herbal that was his greatest achievement but his role as an educator of the common people and midwives in matters of health care: 'I shall do good to my countrymen; yea, them that are yet unborn; for their healths (as well as the now living) have I lost my own . . . I love well and am as willing to help all ingeneous men, though their parts be never so weak: but I hate pride in whomsoever I find it. I now bid farewell for this time. Jan, 2. 1653. Nich. Culpeper . . . '[19]

12

Mysteries of Alchemy & Physick

I believe that alchemy is a pretty kind of game,
somewhat like tricks o' cards,
to cheat a man with charming.

Ben Jonson, 1572–1637

The *Alchemist* by Ben Jonson is a brilliant portrait of the beginning of the 17th century, a time when alchemy was still considered part of medicine and slowly emerging as the forerunner of modern chemistry. In this play, Johnson takes the magic out of alchemy and astrology: he ridicules Subtle, the alchemist who was supposed to turn lead into gold, and the Puritans who wanted to be rejuvenated by chemical medicines, like *aurum potabile*.

After the fall of the Roman Empire the decline of learning was much more rapid and severe in the Roman west than in the Greek east. In the east some knowledge of Hippocrates and Galen continued to be preserved and enlarged by Arabic writers such as Al Rhazi, Ali Abbas and Avicenna. Most of these knew their Hippocrates as well as their Galen well and upheld the tradition of Greek medicine, which later became the source of medical teachings in northern Europe.[1] From the east also came mystical theories about astrology and alchemy such as the codex of Hermes Trismegistus, a new ingredient of seventeenth-century medicine. Hermetic medicine, which had become fashionable among radical spirits, was derived from the sacred Egyptian canon of medicine, named after Hermes Trismegistus, the Greek name of the God Thoth.

The most important proponent of the new school of astrology and alchemy was the eccentric Swiss-German physician, Theophrastus

Bombastus von Hohenheim or Paracelsus, as he called himself
(1493–1541). His medical doctrine was based on the analogy between
macrocosm and microcosm: the human organs corresponded to
celestial bodies, e.g. the heart to the sun. The function of these
organs depended on the constellation of the stars and not, as the
ancients believed, on the composition of the humours. Paracelsus
maintained that man must be a peculiar entity, developed from
the seed created by God. He also believed that God, the creator of
life, disease and death had provided man with remedies, specific in
their virtue and antidotal to certain diseases. Paracelsus popularised
opium and his school introduced a battery of new drugs, mostly
'chemical' if not alchemical. These were metals, extracts, elixirs and
distillates.

The appearance of Paracelsus challenged traditional medicine.
His rebellious followers were opposed to the authoritarian Galenic
tradition of humours but fought for the method of patient observation and experiments: cures must be found by experiment and
experience rather than logical deductions according to the codex of
Hippocrates and Galen.[2] The Paracelsians claimed that all creatures
were composed of four elements: earth, fire, air and water and that
the spirit of life can be detected in sulphur, mercury and salt. They
had a simple unified theory that these elements of life could be
reduced to a crystalline quintessence and believed in the healing
power of *aurum potabile*, liquified potable gold, as the heal-all and
life elixir. Paracelsus' medical doctrine also included the concept
of sympathy and thereby became the forerunner of homeopathy.
The dogma of Paracelsus not only included alchemy but also a
fair bit of astrology. The aim of the alchemists was to discover
the transmutation of the baser metals into gold and silver and the
means of prolonging life and curing diseases with metals and their
salts. Paracelsus and the alchemists promoted the idea of separation
and purification of the active substance by distillation to achieve
the *'quinta essentia'* and toiled with alembics and salamanders,
distilling, subliming and calcining.

Culpeper undoubtedly was influenced by this knew thinking, but
he was sceptical towards the idea that every evil should be treated
with minerals or metals. He tried to develop a working compromise
between the doctrines of Galen and Paracelsus, or as his friend and
collaborator William Ryves wrote: 'He was not only for Galen and
Hippocrates, but he knew how to correct and moderate the tyrranies
of Paracelsus.'[3]

A personal comment reveals his opinion: 'Preacher Mr. Thomas Fuller, in writing such base and scurrilous language against that famous man who the world is so much beholding and indebted to: Paracelsus whose name will ever be deer to posterity, though the papists threw all their dirt they could in his face because he was a protestant, and Mr. Fuller raked it up again and threw it upon his ashes.'

Culpeper adopted a number of very fruitful ideas from Paracelsus and his followers such as an opposition to polypharmacy: 'Look upon one of Galens apothecaries shops . . . so many simples are in one composition, that they hinder one anothers operation.' Culpeper was thus sympathetic to Paracelsus and shared his critical view about contemporary medicine, but he did not adopt his 'divine alchemy', his concept of therapy. The treatise *'Aurum potabile'* advocating 'chymical medicines', and attributed to Culpeper, was spurious. It is therefore misleading to call him the 'English Paracelsus'.

Seventeenth-century medicine was a boiling pot of many ingredients, but the mainstream of orthodox teachings of medicine were firmly oriented towards the classical Greek humouralistic teachings of Hippocrates and Galen. To them, health was nothing more than the result of the harmonius mixture of the humours and innate heat. 'Most of my art of physic I owe to, the great Greek physicians Galen and Hippocrates. These men thought of everything in nature as purposeful. Besides, a reverent study of the Creator teaches you more than anything. The best physician is also a philosopher and a healer of the soul and should profess psychologie,the knowledge of the soul.'

We have to view Culpeper from the stage of contemporary medicine. In the early 17th century ancient Greek concepts of medicine had not been seriously questioned for centuries and by Elizabethan statutes of 1570 the teachings of Hippocrates and Galen had been appointed to be the official textbooks of the lectures in medicine at Cambridge. It is significant that Hippocrates and Galen, together with the Arabs Mesue and Avicenna, adorned the title page of the first edition of the *London Pharmacopoeia* of 1618.

The core of conventional medicine in the early 17th century was based on Greek, Arabic and Roman codices which go back to Hippocrates (460 BC) who was universally venerated as the 'Father of Medicine'. He and his disciples proposed that the body was composed of four humours: blood, phlegm, yellow and black bile. These originally corresponded to the four primary elements, fire, earth, water and air which were governed by the temperatures: hot, cold, wet and dry. Health was the balanced state of the four humours and temperatures and disease was defined as a disturbed balance, as something hostile to nature. Diagnostic clues could be found in the colour of urine or the hue of the patient's skin, for each humour was thought to be characterised by a distinctive colour.

The foremost apostle and innovator of Hippocratic medicine was Galen whose ample writings on anatomy, the humoural theory of diseases and principles of treatment were strictly adhered to in the 17th century. Claudius Galen (130–200 AD) was born in Pergamon, Greece and educated in Alexandria. He became physician to gladiators whom he followed to Rome, where he established himself as a very successful practitioner and personal physician to the emperor Marcus Aurelius. At the time Galen was a pioneer who introduced new thinking to medicine. Among other things he introduced a classification of herbal medicine in terms of their reaction with the patient's humours. Galen wrote 500 treatises mostly devoted to medicine, anatomy and philosophy. His anatomical knowledge was obtained from the dissection of animals, including monkeys.

Galen reminds us of Culpeper in that he waged war against his contemporary physicians. He complained that they were not motivated by love for truth but by greed and lust and desire for political power. 'They are ignorant, pretend to admire Hippocrates but they do not follow him.' The early Christians of Rome respected Galen who praised their valour, temperance and justice, virtues he himself extolled. One of the reasons why Galen's teachings for many centuries continued to be compatible with Christianity was his pious sentiments towards the Creator.

In matters of materia medica or medicines Galen's authority was not so high as that of another first century Greek physician in the employment of Nero – Pedanius Dioscorides, the greatest herbalist of all times. Culpeper, in his *English Physitian*, cites him 26 times, before Galen, 17 times. In addition, Matthiolus, the Italian 16th-century commentator of Dioscorides, is mentioned 13 times. The Roman naturalist Gaius Plinius was the second most important writer in matters of herbal medicines.

From Galen's classification comes the connotation of a 'simple', meaning a herb which possesed a single quality such as heat or moisture. By extension, it came to mean one of the plant constituents in a complex prescription. This system was strictly adhered to in the contemporary herbals of Gerard, Parkinson and Coles and can also to a certain extent be traced in Culpeper's *English Physitian* of 1652. Here we read: 'All the violets are cold and moist while they are fresh and green, and are used to cool any heat or distemperature of the body, either inwardly or outwardly, as inflammations in the eyes.'[4]

Hippocratic-Galenic teachings had become a rigid dogma which paralysed development in medicine for 1600 years. We can compare the situation in medicine to the holy dogma of the Catholic church: any attempt to challenge these rules was heresy and resulted in punishment enforced by the church or by the worldly arm of the king. This is not surprising since it had been the prerogative of the church to censor and supervise health care in Britain. In London this role had been taken over by the Royal College of Physicians but in the provinces this was still applicable at the time of Culpeper. License to practise by the physician was granted by the bishops.

Since Galen was regarded as the epitome of medicine it was the ambition of Culpeper to explain his principles to everybody. This he did in the 1652 publication of *Galens Art of Physick,* a book which is composed of 100 chapters dedicated to the afflictions of all parts of the human body, the symptoms and the cures. The principle is explained in chapter 89: 'Cure'. Galen: 'The indication for cure is evacuation and alteration. Alteration is cooling the heat of the humour by cool medicine. This taketh away the effect, but the cause is taken away by evacuation as bleeding, sweating or clysters, or drawing the humors to another place as by blisters and the like.' Drawing the humours to another place was also called derivation.

A nice example of this is given by Culpeper's contemporary, John Evelyn, when he described the 'pulling of the distemper or offending humour away from the site of injury'. In 1646 when travelling in Italy he wrote:

> I was so afflicted with an angina and sore throat, that it had almost cost my life. After all the remedies Cavalier Veslingius, chief professor here, could apply, old Salvatico (the famous physician) being called made me be cupped and scarified in the back in four places; which began to give me breath, and consequently life; for I was in the outmost danger; but God being merciful to me, I was after a fortnight abroad again . . . [5]

(Reading this account it becomes clear that God was certainly merciful to poor Evelyn, who thought he had contracted his throat infection by drinking too much wine chilled with snow. The Veslingius mentioned here was the author of the anatomical treatise, 'Anatomy of the body of man', which Culpeper translated and edited in 1654.)

Although Culpeper adopted and admired many of the principles of Galen he certainly developed his own ideas which he not only presented in his *English Physitian* but also in *Galens Art of Physick*. It is typical for Culpeper that this book not only contains the teachings of the great Greek physician but also his own comments and ideas, often quite different from those of Galen. This is evident from comments he makes in chapter 89: 'It seems that Galen here minded an antipathetical cure, in which his rules are good. There is another way of cure which we call sympathetical, which is done by strengthening Nature in general and part of the body afflicted in particular. Of this and the reason for it everyone that is fit to give physick may see in my English Physitian.'[3] The idea of strengthening nature and helping it to repair damage was a new concept.

This definitely implies that Culpeper was ahead of his time since he prefers to build up the defences of the body by gentle herbal cures, diet and exercise rather than by applying the weakening and destructive procedures of bleeding, blistering and purging. To us today this seems quite reasonable and logical, but at the beginning of the 17th century it was anathema to question bloodletting and purging, the cornerstones of school medicine.

The physician's role was essentially to participate in a battle to restore nature and to find out which humours were wanting or in excess. The physician had to diagnose the disease in term of its humoural imbalance and match it with the appropriate drug to achieve the normal state. Each drug was assigned a special virtue on a scale of four: 'hot and moist in the first degree . . . cold and dry in the second or third degree etc.'

'Health is the state of the body according to nature and disease is the unnatural state. Since nature is purposeful and solicitous for the good of the creature, she does her best to restore unnatural states to their healthy condition. The function of the physician is simply to cooperate with her. The physician must preserve what is according to nature, and eliminate what is not.'

Culpeper advocated exercise, not only in 'Health for the Rich and

Poor by Diet without Physick' but also in his *Directory for Midwives*. These recommendations must be regarded as extremely modern since the value of diet and exercise in our days of jogging and cholesterol watching are being properly appreciated and proven by large-scale population studies. With this in mind it is fair to say that Culpeper in the seventeenth and eighteenth century saved more lives than the collected assembly of recognised and learned physicians using conventional and dangerous methods of treatment such as boodletting, vomiting and purging.

The principle of healing by exercise is further elaborated for people with 'Coldness of moisture, softness of pulse and fearfulness of mind. Much exercise is very convenient for such bodies. I suppose there were but few troubled with this infirmity in the Spartan Commonwealth in Lycerges his time. The rashing and cleaning boys is good physick for them'. The 'sanguine, cholerick, melancholy and phlegmatic: much exercise is very healthful for them unless they love their laziness better than their health'.[4]

The importance of diet is clearly presented in Culpeper's 'Health for the Rich and Poor by Diet without Physick.' Here he wrote:

> What is meant by sober life I intend such an exact quantity of meat and drink, as the constitution of the body allows of in reference to the services of the mind and body. In reference to the services of the mind, because such as lead a studious life, ought not to eat so much, as such as lead a laborious life. Although the matter of this sober life or diet be mainly conversant about meat and drink, yet it forbids excess in all other things called not natural. Youth and age require different quantities . . . It is best for students to use a good quantity of bread with their meat . . . keep as much as may be from the view of dainty feasts and banquets. Sober life mitigates evil influences of the planets and so by the very same rules it as much increases the good and this is a terrestrial paradise to him that useth it far exceeding Parkinson's Garden of Delight.

Certainly these ideas must be regarded as radical and modern in a time when the consequences of overeating meat were all too common. A large number of people – at least in the upper classes, from whom we know best – suffered from diseases induced by overeating meat such as gout, kidney stones and strokes. In this context it is significant to call attention to the fact that the word 'meat' was used synonymously with food. Drink was predominantly ale for young as well as for old. Ale, brown beers and sweet wine are also known to be implicated with *arthritis urica* or gout.

Culpeper does not mind criticising authorities: 'Great men do often lie, which is probable, and so did Aristotle in his Physic: therefore it is in vain to defend their error.'[6] Culpeper was not alone in his criticism of Galen. Francis Bacon called Galen mean-spirited and vain, and held him directly responsible for the conservatism of doctors. Culpeper's medical ideas were a mixture of conventional Greek teachings, folklore and astrology with the addition of some of the new Baconian experimental approach which he describes as: 'Experience is worth more than tradition ten thousand times told over'. Culpeper's motivation in his medical writings was once expressed as: 'Truly my own body being sickly, brought me easily into a capacity, to know that health was the greatest of all earthly blessings. .... I cannot built my faith upon author's words. But labour to be able to give reason for everything. Reason makes a man differ from a beast.'

Culpeper was capable of describing special features of diseases. The introduction to 'The Anatomy of the Body of Man' also contains an example which shows that Culpeper was not a slave to Galenism, but that he had ideas from other sources: 'It is not hard for a man trained in the school of Xermes (xermetical philosophy being far more ancient than Galen's method) to prove that the life in health and disease lies in the temper of their bodies. A man must know in what part of the body a disease lies and the place also, before he knows how to remedy it. I would willingly teach Galenists if they were not too proud to hear.'[7] This principle of actually trying to localise the disease process is at variance with the more general and vague Galenic concept of changes of composition of humours and temperament. Culpeper lends support to this concept of the cause of disease or pathology with his description of pulmonary tuberculosis: 'Things expelled from the lungs are like the parts afflicted, as when such as are troubled with the consumption of the lungs spit out such filth as resembles the flesh of their lungs.'[3] Similarly he gives the first candid description of severe dysentery (membraneous colitis), suffered by his son: 'You may remember that not long since there was a raging disease called the bloody flux, the College of Physicians not knowing what to make of it, called it the plague of the guts, for their wits were at ne plus ultra about it. My son was taken with the same disease, and the excoriations of his bowels was exceeding great; myself being in the country was sent for up, the only thing I gave him was mallows bruised and boyled both in his milk and drink, in two daies (the blessing of God being upon it) it cured him, and here to shew my thankfulness to God in communicating it to his creatures, leave it to posterity.'[4] And in another treatise: 'as it was the last epidemical disease in London when people with their excrements voided things like the skins of their guts.'

Culpeper in his wide scope of medicine also had a good grasp of mental health. The idea of a soul as part of the body fluids was considered materialistic and anathema to puritan christians. Culpeper revealed his view on mental disease thus:

'Madness is a disease of the body, neither it is unknown that folly is a disease of the mind and yet it is epidemical at this time, the more is the pity. It is the body that afflicts the mind, for it is absolutely impossible the mind should afflict the body, the mind being aetherical, immortal and in no way subject to corruption. The mind of man considered alone by itself knoweth all things, but being entangled in the body, and darkened by its cloudiness and infirmities, it can see nothing without the have and help of the body. I hope you see by this time how beneficial the knowledge of the anatomy of a mans body is to the rectification of the endowments of his mind, indeed to his whole wellbeing both in this world and that to come, if he mind virtue here, and intend to inherit happiness hereafter.' This means that Culpeper subscribes to the concept that all ills emanate from the 'corruption of the body', therefore it is essential to have a good knowledge of it. 'If a disease has invaded the spirits, and that is the quickest way to kill a man, carry a urinal full of piss to the doctor and he will say he ails nothing. The reason is no digestion found in the urine, because the disease seized not the body but the spirits.'

As revealed in his *Midwifery* Culpeper's view on the circulatory system upholds the conventional concept by Galen and Riolan although he must have been aware of Harvey's discoveries and Veslingius' more modern description, which he himself translated:

'The heart itself, which is the prince of all bowels, and the fountain of vital heat and spirit, by whose flourishing the creature flourisheth and by whose languishing it languisheth and by whose failing it dies. I call it the fountain not of the primoginial heat produced by the substance of seed, but of the influential heat which is taken from nourishment, or drawn by blood. It communicates to the whole body by the arteries. The vena cava fills its ventricles and this causeth a perpetual motion of blood to the heart. For the same very end nature hath placed the veins as companions to the arteries, that they might readily receive what might be administered to the emptying of the heart for the exact knowledge of which our age is beholding to William Harvey.' – Culpeper disagrees with this: 'I confess I differ in opinion from him (Veslingius) in some few particulars, and but in a few, especially where he makes the heart the fountain of blood, as also the veins that carry it, wherein it is apparent that he drank too deep of Aristotles spittle: I confess I passed it in silence.'[6]

In silence Culpeper bypasses Harvey, the eminent contemporary physician and originator of the the concept of circulation. He prefers not to acknowledge his name and puts the blame on Aristotle. Culpeper simply despises physicians although he denies this in his writings.

In the 17th century we repeatedly hear about the 'mystery of physick' and the 'mystery of pharmacy'. Culpeper tells us: 'The College of Physitians forbiding the mystery (as they call it) of physick from you. Hiding the ground of physick from the vulgar is the reason'.[3] What is meant by this? An explanation is given in King James' I motivation to separate apothecaries from druggists and spicers: 'Grocers are but merchants; the business of the apothecary is a mystery; wherefore I think it fitting that they should be a corporation of themselves . . . Very many empiriks and unskilful and ignorant men do make and compound many unwholesome, hurtful, deceitful, corrupt, and dangerous medicines. To the great peril and daily hazard of the lives of our subjects.' This, in a way, meant that apothecaries were to uphold a secret art.

It is noteworthy that Culpeper the astrologer did not think of medicine and pharmacy as something mystical at all; therefore it is wrong to believe that Culpeper was a mystical quack who tried to use supernatural forces in his practice. No, he regarded medicine, pharmacy and astrology as very realistic, a science or craft that could be learned by anybody ambitious and responsible. Culpeper very much thought of himself as being in touch with the modern age and was averse to superstition:

> If superstition had not been the father of tradition, as well as ignorance the mother of devotion, this herb (St Peter-wort) as well as St. John's wort had found some other name to be known by; but we may say of our forefathers as St Paul and the Athenians, I perceive that in many things you are too superstitious; yet seing it is come to that pass, that custom having gotten possession pleads prescription for that name. I shall let it pass and come to the description of the herb.[4]

Finally, Culpeper's general concept of medicine is revealed by him when he says: 'Nature is liberal to provide for the necessities of the poor and has sent forth many matters of medicaments, that may be found everywhere and with little art may be prepared.'[8]

> My art of physick I profess is such that we should first of all not do any harm. Let us not overwhelm our patients with crowds of drugs. Like Hippocrates says: We must subtract from what abounds, and add to what is wanting. We follow Galen's art of healing by insisting on contraries for all cures are performed by contraries. I only differ in opinion about the universal cure of blood-letting Galen advocates. This cannot be wholesome and it may deplete the body of nourishing and solicitous juices. According to our learned physicians there is no distemper that should not be treated by bleeding, purging or vomiting. If somebody bleeds from haemorrhoids, the nose or spits blood they say do not stop it, let it be, this is the way of the body to rid itself of sickness. But bloodletting, makes you weak and swooning. Is our blood not containing vital spirits and nutrition, why deplete the body of this precious fluid? Most doctors speak in favour of evacuations, to release distempers from the body. Is this achieved by bloodletting, purging, vomiting and expectorations? Can we rid our bodies of the evil humors, offensive phlegms and black bile by these simple measures? And what if disease really is not the result of an abundance of bad fluxes but rather, a deficiency, a lack of something which we could replenish? Galen himself said

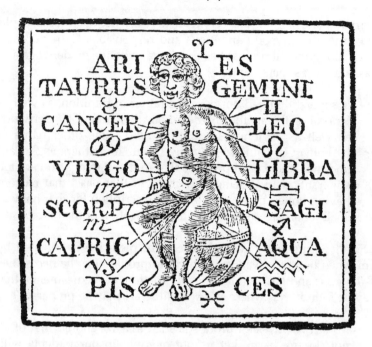

Figure 3. **Anatomy of a Man's Body as Governed by Celestial Signs**
Source: Riders's British Merlin, London, 1763.

that purgative physick is contrary to nature, takes away some of our best spirits, and consume the very substance of our bodies.

With the introduction of experimental science and medicine based on observation of the patient and the development of pathology, the teachings of Galen finally disappeared over the following centuries. Today the only remaining fragments can be found in pharmacy terms like 'Galenic formulation'. The overthrow of Galen in medicine left Hippocrate's reputation in many respects untouched and until today we admire Hippocrates not because of his medical teachings in anatomy and physiology but rather because of the high standards of his medical ethics. We regard Hippocrates as the ideal of the compassionate, discreet and selfless doctor.[1] Today medical students in many parts of the world (including Kuwait) still profess the Hippocratic oath at their graduation ceremony.

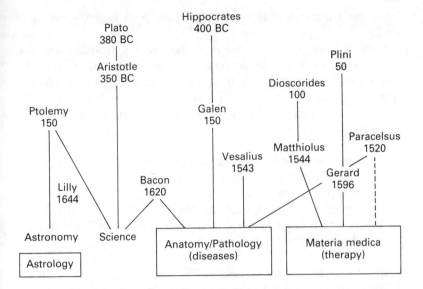

Figure 4. Chart Showing the Source and Development of Culpeper's Ideas

One of the most important applications of astrology was the practice of medicine. The planets possessed the qualities, heat, cold, dryness and moisture corresponding to the terrestrial elements, earth, fire, water and air. These forces were transmitted to the human body by the Galenic humours, blood, bile (choler), black bile (melancholy) and phlegm. The influence of astrology on medicine was intimately associated with the firmly accepted tenets of Galen's humoral pathology. And the signs of the zodiac corresponded to various organs as displayed in the 'zodiacal man'.

Seventeenth-century medicine still heavily depended on astrological assumptions. Many leading physicians like Richard Forster, president of the Royal College of Physicians accepted the importance of astrology and traces survived even in the practice of the famous William Harvey, who prescribed a mixture to be taken 'every new and full moon'. Culpeper firmly believed in the rational use of astrology which he thought to be superior to uroscopy of the accredited physicians: 'None should have just occasion to say of us astrolgers that we do as physitians vulgar practice is, when they judge of piss . . . Yet mistake me not, I do not deny but such whose daily experience is to judge waters and usually judge a hundred in a day may know something by them: If anything may be known by urine, I am sure it is by art. Put them both together, *vis unita fortior.'*

Culpeper was very interested in the process of vision and the diseases of the eye. His interest was so great that he actually participated in the dissections of sheep and cat's eyes, as already mentioned. In trying to explain why a cat sees better at night he came up with the following explanation based on his own observations:

1. The crystalline humour of the cat's eye was far clearer.
2. The iris was much clearer.
3. The optic nerve in the cat was much bigger.
4. The optic nerve of the cat had two originals at a great distance from each other, the one from the cerebrum of brain and the other from the cerebellum.

In his supplement to the *London Dispensatory* Culpeper mentions a large number of 'opthalmics' or 'medicines appropriated to the eyes'. There are herbs such as Eye-bright, seeds of Oculus Christi, Rew, Ivy-leaves, Tormentil and Marigolds; also woman's milk and Hogs-grease. Another example of medicines that 'strengthen the visive vertue' is 'Goats Liver which conduceth much to make one see in the night'. To-day we can explain the therapeutic value of this medicine on the basis of its content of vitamin A.[9]

Medicine during Culpeper's lifetime was still largely under the influence of scholastic teachings, and the acceptance of ancient principles based on the teachings of Greek and Roman scholars. Alchemy was both new and vitalising, but also a confusing new element; empiricism in its true sense of the word only slowly gained ground in medicine. Science slowly emerged by the work of such men as Francis Bacon and William Harvey, men who relied on experimental proof and oberservation rather than theory and tradition.

There is no doubt that Culpeper was a serious man who had the ambition to embark on a new path not because of family tradition, but because of an inborn creative passion to seek the truth, to achieve and to heal.

13

Printed Matters

We skim off other men's wits, pick the
choice flowers of their tilled gardens to set
out our own sterile plots. We lard our lean
books with the fat of other's works.

Robert Burton, 1577–1640

One cold, drizzly afternoon in the November of 1653 Peter Cole, his publisher, came visiting and found Culpeper depressed and lying in bed. He was not his usual self, not sitting at his desk and writing. Cole sensed that something was wrong. He heard him breathe heavily.

'Look what I brought for you, the latest books in medicine from the Continent and among all the learned Latin texts here are two intended purely for your entertainment.' He had brought *The compleat Angler* by Isaac Walton and the *Pennyless Pilgrimage* by the waterpoet, John Taylor.

Cole said to him: 'I advise and counsel you, for at least an hour after dinner, to sit and recreate yourself with reading some light and and merry matter, abandoning cares and fancies out of your mind. This will bring you pleasure, your mind being relaxed and wonderfully comforted.'

When he returned to Spitalfields after a week Cole asked Culpeper what he thought of *The compleat Angler*.

'Isn't it a delightful tale of innocent pleasure combined with useful observations?'

'Yes, it appears to be a nice mixture of verses and thoughts. It carries the message of feeling sluggish, sitting for hours near a brook and listening to Nature's tale of wind and water, birds' song and waiting for the fish to bite. But, to be honest with

147

you, it does not appeal to me at all. My friend, Mr. William Lilly, the astrologer, used to be very fond of angling. I admire people like him who can relax, sit and reflect; but it is not my style. I am too restless, I am a man of quick mind and ceaseless action.'

'You being a wise man and a man of experience in Nature. What did you think of Walton's tale about the eel being created out of mud and not by spawning? Is this not contrary to all rules in the animal kingdom? How can an animal be conceived out of water and dirt?'[1]

'No, I think that is quite possible. There are many mysterious things on Earth, things that are governed by the stars. The eels are the offspring of Jupiter and I am not alone in this opinion. The famous John Gerard and Matthias Lobel have clearly reported that animals can be hatched out of barnacles, and conceived of rotten planks and mud, such as the sea-geese. Let me show you what Gerarde wrote in his book.'

Culpeper went to the next room which was filled with books and brought a big folio in yellow vellum, opened it and read: 'At the end of our history of plants, to end with one of the marvels of this land (we may say of the world), there are found in the north parts of Scotland certain trees whereon do grow shells of white colour, wherein are contained little living creatures which in time of maturity do open, and out of them grow those little living things which falling into the waters do become fowles which we call barnacle geese.'

Gerard also writes about similar things from Lancashire: 'In short space after it comest to full maturition and falleth into the sea where it gathers feathers and groweth to a fowle bigger than a mallard and lesser than a goose.' Also on the Kentish shores and on the rocks of Guernsey and Jersey he observed limpits on planks and rocks with 'living things like a bird'. But at the end he says: 'I dare not absolutely vouch in every circumstance. I leave it to further consideration.'[2]

'I myself have not had time to search for these miraculous things because I cannot leave my work and I am too weak.'

'But isn't it blasphenous to maintain that geese are created out of mud and sunshine?'

'No, not at all, in the end our Lord has created all of us and every living creature out of dust and mud and to dust we will return, as it is said in the Bible. That is the story of barnacle geese. I know my time is limited and I have to get on with my work. I shall never be content until I have completed all the parts of the English Physitians' Library.'

All his life he was busy writing. Between patients and house calls he rushed upstairs to pen down some ideas about the secrets of medicine and therapeutics. He was not content to work only on one text, but simultaneously translated anatomy, medical texts and wrote down his own ideas.

Culpeper certainly was a man with an encyclopaedic mind and the ambition to reform the whole system of medicine. He wanted to get to the bottom of things, to explain and give reasons. It is not surprising therefore, that he devoted much time and effort to the 'basic sciences of medicine'. In the 17th century this still was mainly anatomy. Culpeper translated three anatomical treatises, which constituted a great contribution to English medicine.[3,4]

The first was John Vesling's '*Syntagma anatomicum*'. Culpeper's English translation already appeared during his lifetime in 1653. On the title page he gave the following declaration: 'The Anatomy of the Body of Man; wherein is exactly described every part thereof, in the same manner as is commonly shewed in public anatomies. And for the further help of young physitians and chyrurgions, there is added very many copper cuts, far larger than is printed in any book written in the English tongue. Also explanations of every particular expressed in the copper plates.'

Johan Vesling, a German from Westphalia, was professor at the University of Padua from 1632–1648. He was also director of the botanical gardens there and made scientific journeys to Canada and the Orient to study botany. The chair of anatomy at Padua had been made famous by the founder of modern anatomy, Andreas Vesalius, and later William Harvey. Vesling's work was very popular and also appeared in German and Dutch. 'The Anatomy of the Body of Man' was a translation of the 1647 edition which had been printed in Padua, it was adorned with 24 copper plates, faithful copies of the originals which were also used in the English edition of Riolan's book. It is interesting to note that this is the first and only book which, during Culpeper's lifetime, contained illustrations; his most important work, the *Herbal*, was without illustrations.

The next to appear was his translation of Jean Riolan's *Enscher-eiridium Anatomicum et Pathologicum* possibly from the Leyden edition of 1649. Riolan was physician to the Queen and a professor of both anatomy and botany at Paris. He met William Harvey in London and disputed with him the concept of the circulation of blood; later he refuted it in his book. The title page of his work began: 'A sure guide; or the best and nearest way to Physick and Chyrurgery; that is to say the arts of healing by medicine and manuel operation. Being an anatomical description of the whole body of man, and its parts with their respective diseases. Englished by Nich. Culpeper, Gent and W.R. Doctor of the Liberal Arts, and Physic. London, 1657.'

When this translation came out, Culpeper was dead. The identity of W.R., the coauthor, is uncertain. The British Museum catalogue suggests that he was W. Rand, but he is more likely to be W. Rowland who also helped with the translation of Riverius' *Practice of Physick*.

The last of the three anatomical translations was the English version of the Danish anatomist Thomas Bartholin's *Anatomia ex Caspari Bartholini parentis institutionibus* which had appeared in a number of editions. We know from the 1651 *Directory for Midwives* that Culpeper had started working on Bartholin's 'Anatomy' a long time prior to its final publication in 1668. It was probably finished by Abdiah Cole since it included also two epistles of Johannes Walaeus concerning the motion of chyle and the blood, which incorporated the modern concept of the circulation (to which Culpeper did not subscribe).

The medical writing of Thomas Bartholinus, the Danish physician and scientist rapidly attracted interest not only on the Continent but also in England. The Latin texts brought from Copenhagen were soon very much sought after by physicians and teachers, and Bartholin's *Anatomy* is mentioned by Samuel Pepys in his diary.[5] The new book of Thomas Bartholin combined the important descriptive features of an atlas of anatomy, showing all the organs of the body, with a description of the function and physiology of different systems.

But all this was only available to the learned classes who mastered Latin. Everybody else could only guess and stare. Therefore Nicholas decided to make a translation. He was probably encouraged in his effort by his printer, Peter Cole, who brought him a copy of Bartholin's work. The offer to make a translation was tempting because he was offered ready money ('for which he paid my husband'); in view of his failing health and his dwindling practice as a physician and apothecary, this seemed a good solution to his pecuniary problems. The English version was published in 1663, together with Abdiah Cole. How much of the *Anatomy* of Riolan and Bartholin was really translated by Culpeper himself cannot be estimated for both were printed after his death.

As we have seen for all his studies of anatomy, Culpeper in his own writings never put forward Harvey's new concept of the circulation of blood. This is evident when reading his *Midwifery*, and the parts concerned with the circulation in the male and female genital organs. The reason might have been that he himself mostly consulted Vesling and Riolan, both of whom never embraced Harvey's teachings. Bartholin, however, was a believer but Culpeper's edition of his work came out thirteen years after his death and it is difficult to know how much he actually worked on it. The other reason might be a voluntary suppression of Harvey's arguments since they came from one of the most outstanding members of the hated College of Physicians.

Culpeper's main printers were Peter Cole and Nathaniel Brook. Cole, who appeared as 'Printer and bookseller at the sign of the printing-press in Cornhill near the Royal Exchange' published most of his important books: the *Dispensatory*, the *Midwifery*, the *Treatise of the Rickets*, the *Herbal*, *Galens Art of Physick* and *The Anatomy of the Body of Man*. Brook was responsible for the esoteric astrological texts such as *The Astrological Judgement*, the *Ephemeris for 1652*, the *Last Legacy* and the *Fall of the Monarchie*.

By the time Culpeper's health failed he had acquired a reputation as a celebrated medical writer whose books sold well. The Coles took advantage of the situation; Abdiah Cole collaborated with Culpeper in his last years and probably was employed to edit and revise the numerous translations of Culpeper. Abdiah Cole (1610–1670?) appears together with Culpeper in a number of translations such as Bartholin's *Anatomy*. He calls himself 'Doctor of Physick' but if or where he graduated is not known. It seems likely that he was a relative of Peter Cole.[4]

How could Culpeper translate and edit the large number of English and foreign books by other authors with illustrations and all? Was Culpeper not a plagiarist? These books appeared long before the introduction of copyright in England and Culpeper always made his own additions. The translation of the *London Dispensatory* included 'many hundred additions which the reader may find in every page marked with this letter A'. Overt plagiarism is stealing work of others *verbatim* pretending that it is one's own and without citing the source. This also happened in the seventeenth century. One example is John Brown's *Compleat Treatise of the Muscles* (1681) which was an exact copy of previous work by William Molines of 1648. The publication did not result in any legal action but a reprimand by James Young.[6]

Culpeper was well aware of the nasty business: 'several men have made objections gainst them (my books). First they object against many additions to the several impressions that have been printed in my books. To which I give these answers: first I seldom made my additions to any of them, unless they were counterfeited (by fellows as like thieves, as pomewater is like an apple), and then I felt myself bound to do something to distinguish my children from their illigimate brood.' In the introduction to a later issue of his *Pharmacopoeia Londinensis* he feels compelled to announce: 'there is a counterfeit edition of this, in which are so many gross errors, that I must say, though it bear my name, it is none of mine, I do disclaim it, there being thirty gross errors in three sheets thereof.'

Culpeper had absolutely no scruples about translating foreign texts without permission. He considered his a new text; moreover he always added a multitude of his own comments so that it looked like a different work. One might wonder how in the seventeenth century it was possible to copy and translate books as freely as this activity took place. But no copyright existed and only the printer could obtain protection against piracy of a book by virtue of its entry in the Stationers' Register. Despite this, pirate editions appeared rather frequently, and particularly of such popular works as Culpeper's *Herbal* and *Midwifery*. Culpeper complained about that when he wrote: 'Observe that there is a conterfeit edition of this book, which goes under my name, but I do disclaim it.'

The pirated editions often were not identical, probably on purpose, in order to disguise them as a new work. A translation of a book from a foreign language was considered acceptable without special authorisation. In the extensive correspondence of T. Bartholin, available in Copenhagen, there are no letters from Culpeper and his name is not mentioned. Therefore it seems that Culpeper did not seek permission for translating Bartholin's *Anatomy*. Criticism of Culpeper's translations would be unworthy for they are the only appearances in English of three of the most popular anatomy books of their time and he deserves everlasting credit for this fact alone.[3]

One of the few English physicians whom Culpeper respected was Francis Glisson, who was for more than forty years Regius Professor of Physic at Cambridge, although he was almost never in residence, as he carried on a busy practice in London. It is possible that Culpeper met him briefly while in Cambridge before he left the University. Culpeper translated his *'Anatomia hepatis'* and his *Treatise of the Rickets*.

It had always been Culpeper's wish to study medicine properly, and he meant properly: it was not just a question of receiving a degree in medicine and the approval by the Royal College of Medicine to practice in London. No, when he wanted to do something it had to be all the way, thorough and intense, for that was his nature.

During his life, with his immense experience from practice, reading and writing, he never called himself 'Doctor of Physick', as so many others with much less knowledge did. In the title of his books he appeared as 'Student in physick and astrology', obviously the permanent student, always in quest of knowledge, never content with himself, demanding the highest possible and impossible goals. After his death many publications appeared under the name of Culpeper, MD.

In the 17th century the distinction between astrology and astronomy was not clear-cut. Not only astrologers but also many scientifically minded astronomers compiled their own *ephemerides* (predictions), partly because of financial gain but also because this was the best way to become known and famous. Tycho Brahe and Johannes Kepler were interested in exploiting their astronomical discoveries. Kepler wrote his own almanacs and Brahe dabbled in medicine. He prepared elixirs and formulae some of which survived in the Danish pharmacopoeia of 1658.

Magic, like sex in our time, was a saleable commodity unlikely to be promoted solely by critical or rational means.[7] Publishing prognostications in almanacs was a major enterprise of astrologers and Culpeper was only one of the large number of compilers flourishing during the 17th century. He published his *ephemerides* for the years 1651, 1652 and 1653 and like the famous Lilly he also had a special issue for the eclipse of the sun in 1652.

Apart from the Bible, almanacs were the most common and influential form of literature in Tudor and Stuart England. They were bought by many people who read little else; they became an important means of education and news long before the advent of newspapers. Basically almanacs of the 17th century contained tables of astronomical and astrological events of the coming year such as movements of planets in the zodiac and details on eclipses and prognostications not only about the weather and harvests, but also about political events, good and evil days and medical notes. A typical feature was also the zodiacal man, a figure which showed organs and parts of the body controlled by the various signs of the zodiac. To all this was added a chronological review of world history. Later a list of fairs was added and blank pages for diary notes.

The sale of almanacs was a very lucrative business not only for the authors but also for the printers and distributors. In the 17th century there were no fewer than 235 authors of these popular publications and in the 1660s sales of almanacs averaged about 400,000 copies annually.[8]

Prognostications of the almanacs were biased according to the inclination of the author and therefore clearly expressed political opinions. Culpeper was an outspoken pro-parliamentarian and against monarchy, which he exposed as tyranny in his: 'Catastrophe Magnatum, or the Fall of Monarchie, A caveat to Magistrates, Deduced from the Eclipse of the Sunne, March 29, 1652'. He held an apocalytic view about the future and predicted the coming of a new age of peace with equal rights for all people when he said: 'Jupiter delights in equality, and so do I.' He predicted that 'The plebeians will rise up; Kingdoms will be changed and beggars will get on horse-back.' In all his publications he fought for the education of the general public, and not only in matters related to health care. Despite these egalitarian principles Culpeper cannot be accused of being a Leveller or early communist, for he stressed his opposition to any 'community of property'.[9]

It is surprising to note that the translation of the *London Pharmacopoeia* did not result in any official protests from the Royal College of Physicians and even passed unnoticed in the annals of the Apothecary Society. *Catastrophe Magnatum*, however, stirred opposition and from the Council of State papers we hear: 'The book published by Mr Culpeper referred to the Committee for Examinations, who are to sent for and examine him thereon, or any other person who have had any hand in its contriving, printing, or publishing, and secure them if they see cause.'[10]

Culpeper not only cared for the sick and wrote popular books about medicine, but also gave public lectures on the art of medicine and astrology. These were recorded in his book *Semeiotica Uranica* (Astrological judgment of diseases).[9] In this book Culpeper makes a statement about epilepsy which is worth mentioning: 'Convulsions are not a disease of the heart but of the braine. The nerves have their origin from the braine, convulsions is a plucking or twitching of the nerves, ergo it is a disease of the braine and not the heart.'[9]

Two Books of Physic appeared in 1656. The text was mainly a translation of the Latin text of John Prevotius but with Culpeper's comments. It seems to be a genuine product. Among other things it contains recipes to facilitate childbirth and afterbirth, such as 'Remedies that expel the secundine'. In the introduction he says:

> Nature is liberal to provide for the necessities of the poor and hath sent for many matters of medicaments, that they may be found everywhere and with little art be prepared. I have followed the expressions of the famous and learned doctor John Prevotius. My intent in publishing books of physick in English is not to make fooles physicians but to help those that are ingenious, rational and industrious. Let me warn thee now, as I have often before that there is great danger in physic if they are not rightly prepared and given in due quantities. And always remember thou shalt give an account to God for all thy actions done in flesh. Therefore when thou hast to do in what concerns the lives of man, do nothing but what thou wouldest do, if thou wert shure the great and dreadful day of judgment were to begin next hour. I shall say no more but this, I am resolved not to give over, until I have published in English whatsoever shall be necessary to make an industriuos, deligent, rational man a knowing physician.

This carefully worded warning probably came in response to the accusations of the physicians that Culpeper did more harm than good and maybe also was a reflection on some incidents of poisoning that actually may have happened after the *London Pharmacopoeia* had become public property. Many medicines in the *Pharmacopoeia* were potentially dangerous whereas most of Culpeper's favourite remedies in his herbal must be regarded as innocuous. Culpeper was careful not to imply that everybody could act as a physician, but only 'industrious, deligent, rational man' (and woman).

Culpeper's School of Physick appeared posthumously in 1659. It begins with a lengthy introduction by his former wife, Alice (who in 1656 had married John Heydon). It contains material which was very alien to Culpeper, like: 'Fragmenta aurea, the first Golden Century of chymicall and physicall aphorisms and admirable secrets', 'The Chyrurgeons Guide' and 'The expert Lapidary or the secret vertues of Stones', 'Phlebotomy displayed', 'The Mystery of the Skill of Physick', and 'Chymical Institutions'. It is noteworthy that none of these subjects have been mentioned in Culpeper's ample literature while he was living and therefore it is very unlikely that this book was his brainchild. In his *Midwifery* Culpeper openly revealed his incompetence in matters of surgical obstetrics and elsewhere, on 'urinary obstruction', he argues against surgery: 'I do not well fancy Galen's remedy of cutting such as have the stone, I think, nay am confident remedies not dangerous to be found for the stone in some of my works.' 'The Chyurgeons Guide' therefore is certainly not by him.

Alice, probably under pressure from her new husband wanted to sell new publications in the name of the famous dead author. She tried every possible trick to make it look like a genuine product, but the sentimental introduction speaks for itself:

'Having an orphan, or posthumus in my protection and being sollicited by divers for the propagation of the publick good in its publication, for its better entertainment, I appear to tell the world it is a legitimate child of Mr. Nicholas Culpeper, my deceased husband. And as I promise you it is the genuine and ingenious off-spring of his brain, so I question not, it will with the rest of his laborious pieces help to blow the trumpet of never dying fame. I need not much endeaver to attest that this tractate is his, for it will evidently appear at first sight, that it is the childe of such a father, which will be commendation enough both for the one and the other, and that is the reason I refused to seek a patron for it, since I know that his bare name will sufficiently serve for a patronage. I follow the new mode of time by disallowing of godfathers, yet the bookseller thought it inconvenient, that this treatise should wander up and down the world without a name, and therefore it is christened The School of Physick. I shall please anyone to cast their affection on this fatherless child, him shall I esteem as my gossip. Expect from me to say no more at present because I willingly cross an old saying: women are never silent till dead. I am in all vertous endeavers for the public good.' signed Alice Culpeper, Nov 15, 1658. 'From my house in Spittalfields, next door to the Red Lion'.

Obviously she was hard pressed to make it look like a genuine product. She did not manage to solicit the patronage of a well-known society man. Instead she asked Culpeper's previous collaborators to add some favourable comments about their former master and friend. A number of them complied and contributed with brief comments such as: 'Mr. Culpeper being truly sensible made it his business not to puzzle his young students with the multiplicity of medicines but only to select and set down such as are most proper choice.' (R.W.) John Gadbury added the nativity of Culpeper and his amanuensis William Ryves wrote a short life of his master – the only one ever written until this day. Jeremiah Borrough concluded with a short prayer but nobody commented about the authenticity of the text.

The book *Aurum potabile* was published as a sensational treatise in the name of Culpeper with the object of making money on its revenues and possibly also to sell an expensive nostrum, something which was very alien to Culpeper. It was probably the brainchild of John Heydon, now married to Culpeper's widow, Alice. The introduction, written by Alice, mentions the collaboration of Drs Freeman and Galstone: 'A treatise touching Aurum potabile or rare Golden Liquor, the true legacy, is a rare cordiall and universall medicine, the perfection whereof was studied out, and attained unto the joynt andeavours of Dr. Freeman and my husband.' Further: 'Dr. Galstone, if all his skill in chymistry, of which the Rosie-Crucian Seraphical illuminated fraternity are the chief masters.' These persons never before or after appeared as co-authors with Culpeper.

These collaborators were friends of Heydon, who was associated with the mystical society of the Rosicrucians and who has been characterised by Ashmole to be 'an ignoramus and a cheat', an opinion in which most of his contemporaries concurred.[8,12]

Aurum potabile is quite obviously spurious. Already in 1655 a pamphlet appeared which questioned its authenticity. It read: 'Culpeper revived from the grave. To discover the cheats of the grand imposter aurum potabile. Here is a woman that cures all diseases with aurum potabile. She has two apple squires both fellow workers, sharers with her, one a gentleman physician, the other called by the name of F. There is a conspiracy in Spitalfields. Obtruding upon Culpers name their pernicious libel. A copy never writ by his hand. This illigitimate libel to injure the dead.'[13]

The majority of titles attributed to Culpeper appeared after his death, but it is not entirely clear to what extent he really was the author or translator. His surviving wife wrote: 'My husband left me seventy-nine books, of his own making or translating into my hand. He also left seventeen books, completely perfected, in the hands of Mr. Peter Cole, for which he payed my husband in his life-time.'[14] This seemed to be an exaggeration.

Already in 1664 Matthew Mackaile, a Scottish physician, suspected that it was very unlikely that Culpeper in addition to the fifteen books which were published during his lifetime would have been able to write the manuscript of another 96.

Mackaile wrote: 'Let the sober and judicious reader judge of the probability of this, considering that he had not above nine years for this work and his astrological studies also (he stopped to write in the year 1648 or 1649 and died in 1654).'[15]

The best judge of Culpeper's bibliography is the author himself, who shortly before his death in the introduction 'To the Reader' tells us:

'Some have objected against my writing books in English. First, I answer, that I have so many precedents for that in French, Italian and Greek authors; as I question not; but will fully satisfy all honest souls. Second, I had so much succes in them already published, that I shall never be content until I have compleated all the parts of the English Physitians Library.'

'I have written seventeen books of physick (besides those already published) which will discover to you the whole method of physick, both according to Paracelsus and Galen's practice; I have also to each of the seventeen books made several appendixes, which I have so contrived, that they may be properly inserted into each of the seventeen books in several places in them; which I will undoubtedly do, if any person be so bold as to counterfeit any of my books. But I shall print them alone, if it be not so abused, that none may be compelled to buy anything twice.'[16]

An assessment of Culpeper's production includes 15 books published during his lifetime plus the addition of the 17 'completely perfected' books mentioned by Culpeper and his wife Alice. This would imply 32 titles and if some of the appendices he mentions were published separately it could roughly correspond to the 38 titles collected by Poynter, an astonishing accomplishment, although some of them were only short tracts.

After his death there was an explosion in the number of new and re-issued Culpeper-books. The *Midwifery* in five re-issues survived until 1777 and the *Herbal* appeared in no less than 70 editions until today, the latest in 1983.

After writing all the books about conception, midwifery, childcare and adult medicine the only topic that remained was geriatrics. It is not surprising that he expressed an ambition to cover even this topic: 'I do intend speedily myself to write a treatise of the same, viz. a guide for Old Age.'[11] This never happened, among all the many tracts there is none that specifically addresses this question. Maybe he wanted to postpone it until he was old himself, but that never happened, he died at the age of thirty-eight. On December 30, 1653, eleven days before his death, Culpeper probably wrote his last published sentences:

> 'I shall not trouble the reader further, being my self sick and weak, no way fit for study or writing. But now pleasing myself in viewing those things that were written in my health, with this deligthful thought. I shall do good to my countrymen; yea, them that yet unborn; for their healths (as well as the now living). I have lost my own. And could chearfully (for the good of the English Nation) ever cease to be.'
>
> From my House of the East
> side of Spittle-Fields, near
> London. This 30 of December, 1653.
> Nich. Culpeper.[16]

Culpeper's successors as popular medical writers were Joseph Blagrave (1610–1682) and William Salmon (1644–1713). These authors edited medical books but none of them had the calibre of their predecessor. Blagrave in 1674 published a supplement to Culpeper's original *English Physitian* and the enterprising physician William Salmon (1644–1713) continued Culpeper's work to make the secrets of medicine available to a greater public. He was responsible for a new English edition of the *London Pharmacopoeia*, issued almanacs and published an encyclopaedic herbal with twice-weekly instalments, finally amounting to seven hundred and fifty pages. Salmon was in trouble because of his political inclinations which were that of a radical Whig and similar to Culpeper's.[17]

The last great astrological physician in Britain was Ebenezer Sibly (1751–1799), who combined astrology, medicine and the mystics of freemasonry. Sibly was a prolific writer and besides his own works about occult sciences he edited a richly illustrated and popular collection of Culpeper's medical texts which came out in ten editions between 1789 and 1817.[17,18]

The authenticity of books published with Culpeper as author after 1654 has to be carefully examined. As we have seen Culpeper was a 'star writer' of popular medical books and any title with his name was guaranteed to become a bestseller. Culpeper's publishers were aware of this as well as John Heydon and Culpeper's widow, Alice.

14

Culpeper's Ghost

Vex not his Ghost: O! Let him pass.
Shakespeare (*King Lear*) (1564–1616)

What do we know about the character of Nicholas Culpeper? We can make a comparison with the Roman naturalist Pliny, who was one of the ancient classical Roman authors most frequently cited by Culpeper: 'The laborious Caius Plinius Secundus, who lived in the time of Vespasian, and was suffocated by the sulphurious vapours that came from mount Vesuvius, falling at the time on fire; he through overmuch curiositie to see and finde out the cause thereof, approaching too nigh.'[1]

Plinius obviously had an inquisitive mind and, like Culpeper, was a tireless writer about medicine. He was straightforward, distrusted compound preparations but preferred 'herbal simples' and disapproved of professional physicians.

Plinius died at the eruption of Vesuvius when Herculaneum and Pompeii were destroyed. After having landed at Stabiae in the Gulf of Naples a strong inshore wind prevented him from putting out to sea again; and after a night spent under terrible circumstances – earthquake shocks, tidal waves, and a constant rain of cinders from the eruption – he died of suffocation. Some think that it happened because he was eager to study nature's force as closely as possible and to witness the flow of the burning lava. Was he a victim of science and did he in fact die in the pursuit of knowledge? Others maintain that Pliny sailed to Stabiae to assist friends whose houses lay close to the volcanic mountain and rescue them from the heat and the falling cinders.[2] Nobody knows for certain and we can only guess; his fate was similar to that of Culpeper: he consumed his energy in the pursuit of knowledge and died trying to help others, his patients.

Probably the best description of Culpeper as a person was by William Ryves his amanuensis. He summarised his character and wrote:

Mr Culpeper was in his deportment gentle, pleasing,and courteous. His complexion darkish and swarty. His visage rather long than round. Of a presence not so beautiful as amiable. His hair black and somewhat curling. His eyes piercing. His body a little above medium tending to tallness. Of a spare, lean constitution. In his apparel not exeeding the moderation of one of his degree. Somewat careless. He was of a clear and established judgment. Of an eloquent and good utterance. Of a quick spirit full of swift thoughts and mounting. Of a sparkling ready wit, a gift which does not always speak men fortunate. He was sometimes too much overtaken with deep speculations, though melancholly was somewhat contrary to his nature; whatever he said otherwise of himself: so that it may rather be imputed to the crosses of his life, then to his own disposition. His health was often disturbed with adust choller.

Of religion he had a greater share then most physicians use to have; he had so much zeal as to hate superstition, and was no friend to episcopal innovations. In his counsel he was judicious; of a nimble apprehension, with little difficulty in his dispatches. He was a person of so ready a mind, that he could more learnedly and suddenly dictate his papers for the press, then some that do take the lamp and oyl more studiously to contrive them. When he travelled in discourse concerning a patients disease, his understanding cleared all doubts; neither was it so dark or cloudy as some practioners are, who still create new scruples, for he had the luck (for the most part) to look directly on truth. He was too free-hearted, (if not inclining to prodigality). His nature was both noble and honest. He was an excellent companion, and for the most part of a merrry temper. His mirth, as he was used to say when he was far spent in his sickness, was the best cordial he had left against the consumption of his spirits. He was a despiser of the world. A man confident, not jealous of his fortunes, which better enabled him to bear his misfortunes. As he was so far from covetousness that he cared not who was his purse-bearer, so long as that he wanted not for necessary expenses, he durst trust God's providence with the rest: his mind was surprised with higher mysteries then to stoop to such worldly trifles. He was a person that by his art had such a for-sight of the changes of the times, that few events seemed new to him as he was long before (by his astrologic skill) acquainted with them. He was another Tycho Brahe for his knowledge of the future affaires of state.[3]

Some similarities exist between Paracelsus and Culpeper: both were self-made men with a wounded personality who lost parents during their childhood. They felt misunderstood and aimed their poisoned arrows at the pompous and complacent physicians.[4]

The Scottish surgeon physician-divine Mr. Matthew Mackaile in 1664, ten years after Culpeper's death, published a 40-page treatise entitled: 'Culpeper's Character or, a Character of Mr. Culpeper and his Writings.' It was appended to a book with the title: 'Moffet-Well' extolling the medicinal virtues of the mineral wells in Annandale, Scotland.[5]

Rather than being a description of the characteristic features of Culpeper, it is a polemic pamphlet against a rival author. Most of the text is devoted to biblical quotations which are held against Culpeper and some of his views. Mackaile is surprised that Culpeper, despite his schooling at the University of Cambridge on which 'four hundred pounds were spent, does not have enough knowledge of "chymistrie" to understand the proper meaning of 'Quintessence'. He says:

His chief designs were 1. the acquiring of money from printers, for buying of beer and tobacco and 2. the erecting of the trophees of his own fame, upon the ruins of others. He accuses Culpeper of encouraging women empirics, 'Doctrix', in their ill advised practice, and he gives examples of this. Maybe the most biting critique was that of his astrological concepts where he says: 'You must excuse my not meddling with any thing in his writings which is astrological: For I acknowledge myself not to be sufficiently acquainted with the principle of that art, and therefore do refer him to others. Only I will say this, that if his astrology in medicinals be no better than it (and the astrology of others more famous than he) was in politicks, in the time of the Commonwealth (when Monarchy was said to be eternally exiled from Great Britain, by all the powers of heaven) they will mispend their time, who will take the pains to read.'

As an argument against Culpeper's view that medicinal herbs are governed by stars, Mackaile cites the teachings of the Bible that: 'The stars were not created until the fourth day of creation, which was the day after the creation of vegetables.' (Therefore how can the stars reign over herbs?)

His final crushing verdict is: 'Mr. Culpeper's writings are either other mens writings which he hath translated into English, or collections out of other men's work, which he has deformed with malicious, scurrilous, detracting and railing expressions, and studied to beautifie with some ridiculous and (sometimes) impertinent jests.'

It is not easy to describe the character of a person like Culpeper. We only know bits and pieces about his personal life. Fortunately his medical texts are very revealing and it certainly helps that his style is so personal. One way of coming closer to our aim is to compare him with contemporary medical writers.

One person eminently suitable for such a study is the famous English 17th-century physician Thomas Sydenham (1624–1689). With this in mind we can make the following observations: both came from a genteel background and both men supported Parliament, fought the Royalists in the Civil War and were wounded in battle. Sydenham had a much longer and more formal training including a period at the Faculty of Medicine in Montpellier. He obtained University education both at Oxford and Cambridge (where he received his MD) and became a licentiate of the College of Physicians. Both were fervent writers but Sydenham's books all appeared in Latin and although he was generally acquainted with that learned language he solicited 'the assistance of better latinists than himself in preparing his works for the press'.[6]

That is probably the reason why Sydenham's reputation rose more rapidly abroad than at home. In Holland and Germany he was called the 'English Hippocrates'. Sydenham, however, was not a puritan and a man of the poor and needy like Culpeper. His patients came from the higher classes, he practised in Westminster; and like other fine members of the College of Physicians and their rich patients, he left the city of London during the plague in 1665. We can only guess what Culpeper in this situation would have done had he lived long enough.

Sydenham was a superb clinician. He studied and described diseases as natural objects. In his words: 'I have been very careful to write nothing but what was the product of faithful observation, and neither suffered myself to be deceived by idle speculations, nor have I deceived others by obtruding anything upon them but downright matter of fact.' Both were highly intelligent writers, Sydenham with a cool analytical mind and Culpeper with speculative imagination. Both were innovators and had the strong personality needed to break with tradition.

Sydenham was well-to-do and left money to his heirs. He dedicated his books to well-known authorities. Culpeper died poor and never cared much for money; his works were only dedicated to his patients, ordinary men of the 'English Nation' and to 'The Matron'. He only left manuscripts of books to his widow and daughter, and an immense popularity.

In latter days Culpeper was popular with Rudyard Kipling and the American neuro-surgeon Harvey Cushing. Kipling admired Culpeper's approach to medicine and even seemed to enjoy his irrational trait. In 1928, at a dinner party of the Royal Society of Medicine, he said:

> Isn't it likely that the multitude and significance of the revelations heaped upon us within the past few years have made men in self-defence specialise more and more narrowly? Haven't we been driven headlong to abandon our conceptions of life, motion and matter? Is it then arguable that we may still mistake secondary causes for primary ones? Suppose, then, at some future time when the bacteriologist and the physicist are for the moment at a standstill, wouldn't it be interesting if they took their problem to the astronomer, and in modern scientific language, of course – put to him Nicholas Culpepper's curious question: 'What was the aspect of the heavens when such and such phenomena were observed? And isn't it human that in upheaval men may have carried off each his own cherished prepossession and camped beside it – just as refugees do after an earthquake?'[7]

In the last years of his life Culpeper was a sick man. He complained of it when on January 2, 1653, he wrote: 'I had no patience to go through the work till I am more healthful!' and 'being my self sick and weak, no way fit for study or writing'.[8]

He suffered from a chest wound inflicted during the Civil War and probababy had contracted tuberculosis. He was a heavy smoker and most certainly had chronic bronchitis with cough and breathing problems. It is also very likely that he tried to suppress the cough with syrup of poppies or even opium, which was popularised by Paracelsus. On top of everything else both William Ryves and John Heydon tell us that he drank a lot of 'bad wine'.

We have a scenario with a famous man, an author of bestsellers, an esteemed physician, sitting in his study with shortness of breath, no longer able to see patients and surrounded by Peter and Abdiah Cole and his amanuensis William Ryves, all anxious to have him produce more texts for new books or just to give his name for rapidly conceived writings. The situation reminds me of the last days of the sick Salvador Dali, the famous Spanish artist who was exploited by art dealers to sign mass-produced pictures.

A famous man, known for many books of controversial contents, but exciting the mind of his contemporaries in a time of much tumultous political and spiritual unrest, he lived intensively and short, burning like a candle from both sides, an epitome of his age. It is therefore not surprising that his fame lived after him and his person no doubt was surrounded by a veil of mystery, like a haunted ghost. This was realised by his publishers and his wife, who married John Heydon, an astrologer of questionable reputation.

During his short lifetime Culpeper had become a notability, a writer of bestsellers. This obviously had to do with the popular demand for his kind of texts: easy to understand for most people, cheap and small of the kind of modern pocket books. It also helped that he came from a well-known family and that he was a controversial figure who had received publicity in broadsides. His language was frank, simple and provocative. His books sold like hot cakes and became a financial success. His wife and printers took advantage of the situation and tried to push new sensational titles after Culpeper's death. They used his name for the sake of profit.

One of these books is called: 'Mr Culpeper's Ghost, giving sea-sonable advice to lovers of his writings' (1656); and another is entitled: 'Mr Culpepper's Treatise of Aurum Potabile' (1657). The first was written by Peter Cole, the printer, who published most of Culpeper's work; the second is attributed to Culpeper but is most probably spurious and was printed by a rival stationer, George Eversden.[9,10]

The Ghost-book contains a lot of rather incomprehensible rubbish which reminds us of Kenelm Digby's weapon salve. One example:

> Why not the virtues of a magnetic medicament, dropped into the patients urine, especially the urine remaining warm be carried into the inmost bowels of the body especially the liver, spleen, kidney and bladder by the spirits of those parts which came away in the urine, and when the urine becomes cold, to retire into the body whence they came by vertuel attraction caused by the emenation of the visible atomes that come from those parts in the sick body, through the air into the chamber-pot or urinal, to visit their fellow spirits there imprisoned.

The treatise on *Aurum potabile* (drinkable gold) is purely an advertisement for an alchemical nostrum, which was peddled at a high price.

If we want to evaluate Nicholas Culpeper's contribution we have to take into consideration his impact on the progress of medicine in his own time; it is not correct to accept the stereotypical view of F. Garrison who in his History of Medicine says: 'Old Nicholas Culpeper, the arch herbalist and quacksalver of his time who indulged in a vast amount of scurrilous raillary at the expense of the London Pharmacopoeia of 1618 and 1650, but except for his herb-lore, he was himself only a credulous astrologer.'[11]

Agnes Arber in her book on herbals describes him as 'The most notorious exponent of astrological botany'. This judgment may be understandable from a purely botanical point of view, but certainly does not give him justice as a herbalist and physician.[12]

Obviously Culpeper was a product of his own time in which the medieval tradition of acceptance of the authority of the written word was still supreme. It is therefore not surprising to find that *The English Physitian* includes a vast number of citations of ancient authors. Among others Dioscorides was quoted 26 times, Galen 17 times and Plinius 15 times.

The celebrated William Harvey was no exception. He believed in and venerated the teachings of the classical authors like Hippocrates and Galen. In his meticulous anatomical dissections Harvey several times described features that were at variance with the concepts of Galen. Rather than stating that Galen's anatomical descriptions were in error he preferred to explain this on the basis of a 'physical

Nicholas Culpeper

degeneration of mankind since the time of Galen'. Harvey also initially endorsed the concept of vital spirits of air in the liver and the heart, but in the end he disagreed with the prevailing concept of the cardiovascular system.[13]

Disagreement with erroneous concepts, however, is not enough for progress, an alternative and better solution has to be offered and finally accepted. This Harvey did when he presented structural as well as experimental evidence for the concept of the circulation of blood, from the right side of the heart through the pulmonary circulation and then through the left side of the heart, the aorta and the systemic blood vessels, postulating pores or capillaries in the tissues, structures that were later demonstrated by the Italian anatomist, Marcello Malpighi. Harvey's discovery changed the whole concept of medicine and therefore he deserves international fame.

Culpeper undoubtedly was also an innovator who by questioning authority helped pave the way for new thoughts and principles contrary to all traditions. He once wrote: 'Here I care not greatly if I quote a little of Galen's nonsense in his treatise of the Faculties of Nourishment. He saith they (artichoks) contain plenty of cholerick juice (which notwithstanding I can hardly believe) of which he saith is engendered melancholy juice, and of that melancholy juice thin cholerick blood.'[8] We have to remember that to question the great authorities like Galen and Hippocrates was considered blasphemy.

To use as medicine 'simples', i.e. well described herbs instead of mystical concoctions of numerous compounds of no value, certainly was an achievement. Even if the efficacy of these medicines in the light of critical scrutiny of today is questionable, many of them can be regarded as useful placebos that did no harm and replaced poisonous substances like antimony, lead and mercury and offered an alternative to the dangerous practice of bloodletting.

The other great importance of Culpeper was as the first medical educator in the English language who on a large scale translated standard Latin text into English and who himself published useful information of his own, such as *A Directory for Midwives* and *The English Physitian* (Herbal).

In Britain and the English-speaking world such as the American colonies, Culpeper in a sense was to medicine what Luther was to religion in Germany (as a translator of the Bible). Culpeper certainly left an impact on medicine in the English speaking countries, but he never attained international fame. His importance was not so much for orthodox school medicine but rather as an educator of common people and the heritage of folk medicine. His readers in later years were mostly housewives whose ambition was to look after the welfare of their families.

Culpeper's main enemies were the physicians. He tells us about them: 'The College of Physitians of London some of which are already snarling at me, I love them and fear them alike.' Barbara Griggs aptly describes the situation: 'He was everything they feared, resented, and despised: an upstart with enough Latin and learning to make their ignorance a laughing-stock, an apothecary who dared to practise medicine – and with huge success – in defiance of their statutes, and to crown everything, a self-confessed Puritan and Parliamentarian.'[14]

Culpeper was not alone in his criticism of physicians. Not only puritans shared his views. John Earle (1601–1665), the royalist bishop in one of his epigrammatic assays, 'A mere dull physician', wrote:

His practice is some business at bedside, and his speculation an urinal. He is distinguished from an empiric by a round velvet cap and doctor's gown, yet no man takes degrees more superfluously, for he is Doctor whosoever. He is sworn to Galen and Hypocrates, as university men to their statutes, though they never saw them: and his discourse is all aphorisms. The best cure he has done is upon his own purse, which from a lean sickliness he hath made lusty and in flesh. His learning consists much in reckoning up the hard names of diseases, and the superscriptions of gallypots in his apothecary's shop, which are ranked in his shelves, and the doctor's memory. He is indeed only languaged in diseases, and speaks Greek many times when he knows not. If he have been but a bystander at some desperate recovery, he is slandered with it though he be guiltless; and this breeds his reputation and his practice; for his skill is merely opinion. Of all odours he likes best the smell of urine and holds Vespatian's rule, that no gain is unsavoury. If you send this once to him you must resolve to be sick howsoever, for he will never leave examining your water till he have shaked it into a disease. Then follows a writ to his drugger in a strange tongue. If he see you himself, his presence is the worst visitation. He translates his apothecarie's shop into your chamber, and the very windows and benches must take physic. He tells you your malady in Greek, though it be but a cold, or headache. His most unfaithful act is that he leaves a man gasping. Anatomies and other spectactles of mortality have hardened him, and he is no more struck with a funeral than a gravemaker. Noblemen use him for a director of their stomach, and ladies for wantonness, especially if he be the proper man. If he be single, he is in league with his she-apothecary. His two main opposites are a mountebank and a good woman, and he never shews his learning so much as in an invective against them and their boxes. In conclusion, he is a sucking consumption himself, and a very brother of the worms, for they are both engendered out of man's corruption.[15]

How about the apothecaries? What was the view about their maverick colleague? We can assume that some might have been sympathetic for helping them to understand the Latin text of the *Pharmacopoeia Londinensis* and for his brave stand to bolster their status as practitioners. But Culpeper was already a black sheep when he was an apprentice and working for Samuel Leadbetter. From the Court Book of the Apothecaries' Society we know that in 1643 Mr. Leadbeater, his employer was frequently 'ordered and warned to put away Nicholas Culpeper' and 'warned not to employ Culpeper in the making or administering of any medicine'.[16] When *The English Physitian* (Herbal) appeared he must have lost all remaining sympathies since it was designed to encourage people to help themselves without expensive medicines. A somewhat similar situation happened in Paris where the known physician Guy Patin (1602–1672) published his *'Le médecin charitable'*, a do-it-yourself medical manual. Patin openly opposed the apothecaries and wanted to ruin them.[16]

Culpeper also criticized certain divines: 'I was taxed by some for speaking something against the clergy in my epistle of the first edition. I hope I gave no offence to any moderate nor honest divine for I honour them. The bishops must be pulled down and we up in their places forsooth . . . I confess the country clergy was always more moderate and in the works of Mr. Burroughs and Bridges you shall find such stuff.'[17] Jeremiah Burroughs (1599–1646), called by his friends 'Morning Star', was a nonconformist divine who lived in nearby Stepney and who preached every morning at seven o'clock at St Giles, Cripplegate. He was originally educated at Cambridge and became a minister but was suspended when he refused to follow the directions of his bishop to make Royal announcements such as the 'Book of Sports'. Burroughs had the same radical opinion about the clergy and the King as Culpeper and shared his enthusiasm about teaching the uneducated. Burrough wrote tracts for the people and used the same publisher as Culpeper. When in October of 1646 Burroughs fell from a horse and was badly hurt Culpeper came to look after his friend, but everything was in vain for after a week he fell into a coma and despite all efforts he died.

Culpeper distanced himself from his own aristocratic relatives and the appeal to his cousin William Culpeper in the introduction to his tract *'Catastrophe Magnatum'* was left unanswered. Culpeper did not even enjoy the support of the official Parliamentarians during Cromwell's time. We know that Dr. Jonathan Goddard, the first physician to the Parliamentarian army and friend of Oliver Cromwell, called him 'a foulmouth'd impudent scribbler'.[17] Does this mean that Culpeper was isolated? The answer is yes and no. He lost contact with his colleagues, politicians and family but must have gained tremendous sympathies from the newly developing literate middle class.

John Webster (1611–1682) was a friend from Cambridge who became a minister in 1634 but was evicted from his living because of puritan and non-conformist views. Thereafter in Lancashire he turned to teaching and part-time practice of medicine, and in 1648 enlisted in the parliamentarian army as a surgeon. In 1653 he came to London to be reunited with his old friend from Cambridge. He shared with Culpeper the hope for the long awaited millenium which was believed to be nigh in Cromwell's England; although Webster like Culpeper did not believe that Christ would return in person to reign, he thought that spiritual renewal was imminent. Webster, in 1654, in his *'Academiarum Examen'*, attacked the old-fashioned conservative syllabus of the universities of Oxford and Cambridge and recommended the teaching of astrology in the universities of which he said:

> They have not only sleighted and neglected it, but also scoffed at it . . . I cannot without detracting from worth and virtue pass without a due eulogy in the commendation of my learned and industrious countrymen, Mr. Ashmole, Mr. Lilly, Mr. Booker, Mr. Saunders and Mr. Culpeper and others who have taken unwearied pains for the resuscitation and promotion

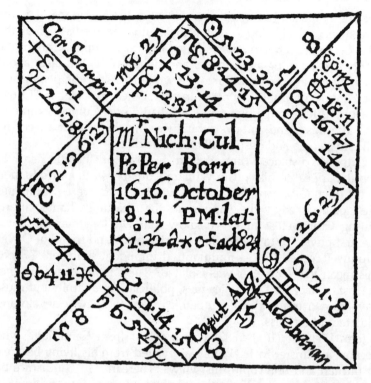

Figure 5.   Horoscope of Nicholas Culpeper by John Gadbury, 1659

of this noble science, and with much patience against many
unworthy scandals have laboured to propagate it to posterity.

John Gadbury (1628–1704) was an admirer of Culpeper and
his ideas and he contributed to the posthumously published
'Culpeper's Art of Physick' where he added a nativity (horoscope)
of his master:

He was full of agility, very active and nimble. His temperature (temperament) melancholy, choleric. Melancholy was an
extraordinary enemy unto him, so great at times, that wanting
company he would his choler afflict him very strangely, even
more than melancholy. He be of an excellent wit, sharp fancy,
admirable conception, and of an active understanding. He was
very eloquent, a good orator, spoke freely and fluently; and I

should speak the truth he was conceited (= full of ideas) and full of jeasts, but the knack of jeasting was so inseperable to him that in his writing things of most serious concernment, he would mingle matters of levity and extreamely please himself in so doing.

He was as free of his purse as his pen, valued not how little he left himself of either, so he obtained his end of doing good to others. He should rise in the opinion of the world. It is well known that he gained his honour by arts and sciences, but chiefly in the knowledge of which he was excellently skilled: and it was purely by the study of practice (of medicine), that he hath left a name behinde him, which will remain until time shall be no longer be.

An abbreviation of the original horoscope was again published in 1792 by somebody signed 'Peter' in the 'Conjuror's Magazine'.[18]

Culpeper's friend, Gadbury, made a remarkable career. He started out as a proletarian Leveller, studied and later practised judicial astrology. He tried to use a more scientific and critical approach in order to reform astrology. Thereby he distanced himself professionally from his former friend Lilly; politically he moved to the right and developed firm Royalist and pro-Catholic sympathies.

In 1658 William Ryves, his amanuensis, concluded about his master:

He was an astrologer, a physician, a great searcher into the secrets of nature and a true lover of the arts, yet such was his modesty, that though he knew so much he made good the saying, he whose own worth doth speak him, needs not speak, his own worth testifies enough of him. He had not many books, but those he had were well selected. He was none of those that persuaded the world he was learned, by getting together a great library, his memory was his Vatican. To conclude he was a better physician to others than to himself.

When he travelled in discourse concerning a patients disease, his understanding cleared all doubts. Neither was it so dark or cloudy as some practitioners are, who still create new scruples, for he had the luck (for the most part) to look directly on truth.

Other friends of Culpeper said: 'His carriage was most mild and temperate by which he love and estimation got. He did not take any excessive gaines but often gave the poor his time and paines.' Joseph Blagrave:

> 'Nothing's impossible, this doctor can
> Heal not the body onely, but the man.'

Thus a picture emerges of a brilliant, impulsive and compassion-ate man, totally devoted to his interests, not caring about trivialities of life. Today we would characterise him as a bohemian genius. Culpeper, however, was no saint; he was restless, arrogant and impulsive, but by no means the charlatan he has been made out to be. His personal style of writing reveals a sense of humour. This was also attested to by his amanuensis William Ryves: 'And sometimes in jeast, as his custom was, he used to say, that there were a certain sort of physicians that were like bishops, they had the keys of binding and loosing, and nothing else.'

He was a devout Christian but he had his misgivings about certain ministers: 'I have heard many ministers that are enemies to astrology. I have known them conversant with them but they durst not look upon the stars for fear they should fall upon their heads for I know no other danger in the art. Astrology is an art which teachest by the book of creatures what the universal providence mind and meaning of God towards man is.'

Convinced about his divine mission he said:

> What remains of us to be done more than by considering the uncertainty of man's life, and how many casualties he is subject to here below, to labour what in us lies to search out the secrets of nature, whereby we may preserve our own lives, the more to glorifie the Maker, and to communicate that knowledge, which by our industry we have obtained, onto the sons of men, our brethren. Doubtless this was that which moved Salomon to make choice of wisdom, accounting riches but dung, and a kingdom, but vanity. Neither did he keep close his knowledge to himself (as too many now a-days do) but he published large discourses. The very same principles first moved me to publish what I knew of the world; and experience witness to me, that the more I reveal that knowledge God has given me to the world, the more he

still teacheth me; and being determined within myself not to give over till I have finished the whole body of physick.

When Culpeper compares himself to King Salomon [Solomon] it cannot be discarded as only baroque rhetoric, but clearly reflects on his personality. Time and again these thoughts are expressed in his writings. Sometimes he is overcome by a philosophical mood and shows great modesty when he concludes: 'Man comes far short of the wisdom of creatures, as I do of the wisdom of Salomon.' In a pessimistic mood about politics and the turmoil in England he philosophically reflects and tells the following fable:

> Take the bees, read but Butler his book of bees, written alto-gether from experience, and you shall see what an admirable martial Common-wealth they keep, how patient in private wrongs. For if you abuse a bee in the field she will not sting you if she can possibly get away without; yet do but affront them at home, then the wrong is public, then if you would save yourself, you must run for it. The truth is no monarchy of men throughout the whole universe was ever compared to them, and yet they never read ethics, and are utterly unacquainted with Machiavellianism, whereas man for all his reading and learning could never frame such a monarch, but may nay, hath undon it self even by Civil Wars (the worst of all other) witnes the Graecians and Roman Monarchies, that I may not spek a word of England.

Culpeper was a proud man but he never pretended to be a physician or doctor, although no doubt his knowledge was far greater than that of many qualified physicians of his time.

> Those that know me rightly, can determine that I was never so inarmoured with that title, but onely to inform my mistaken countrey-men, that it is not the cowl that makes the munk, the shaking of the urinal, the stroking of the beard, hard words, the plush cloak, a large house with a monster in the first room to amaze the patient, but deep grounded reason, and tried experience, that commences a physician.

On the title page of his many books we always read: 'by Nicholas Culpeper, Gent. Student in Physick and Astrology'. The title 'Gentle-man' was never omitted and even to the puritan and parliamentarian

Culpeper the distinction between the gentlemen and a tradesman was an unquestionable fact of life. He was a humble helper of the sick but always aware of his station. Culpeper did not follow the common practice of dedicating books to a person of high rank and standing in order to assure acceptance. There is one exception: he dedicates his *Catastrophe Magnatum* of 1652 to his cousin William Culpeper, Knight and Baronet:[19]

> 'Worthy Sir, before I proceed further, let me crave pardon of your Worship, for these my bold attempts in presuming to dedicate these my weak labours to your Worship, to whom distance of place hath now almost made a stranger, but considering that ingenuity of spirit that was one in your father and flourished in you who are the branch of so noble a root, together with antient familiarity that was between your father and mine, imboldened me after I had converted a few idle hours into study, and having brought forth to birth that what then I conceived, I present it at your Worships feet: I hope there is nothing in it unbeseeming the name of Culpeper, if there be failings in it they are not more than what we are all subject to. The ingenuity of your Worship, I know be such, that you will not only passe by my boldness in dedicating it to you, for that objection our alliance in blood may take off.'
>
> 'I hope your Worship will expect no flattery in this epistle, there being non in the book: if you accept the book I shall thinke myself happy and I am confident those of our blood will hardly degenerate, it was a notable expression of Plato.'
>
> 'Though it has been neer upon 15 years since I saw your Worship; yet I have often heard of you, both by master Thomas Culpeper and master Whitfield who are both our kindred. The truth is there arose a question within myself wether I should dedicate it to your worship or not. Your Worships friendly acceptance of it shall be such a favour to me as I shall never forget, indeed I have so much the blood of Culpeper in me . . . '[20]

It was wishful thinking to assume that William would be flattered and happy to have this doomsday treatise presented to him. Culpeper certainly made a mistake, and in the future no more dedications, except 'to the common people of England', appeared.

Culpeper had a surly and vindictive disposition and in the midst of his anatomical description he wrote:

When the yard stands a few superficial veins and arteries are visible to the eye. These are the parts common both to the yard and also to the rest of the body, which also I have been somewhat large about, yet I cannot account it tedious, because it conduceth to the teaching of knowledge to my countrymen and women, who have been too long reined in with the bridle of ignorance by physitians that so they might be better ridden by them. Our physitians serve the commonality of this nation, viz. hide all from them they can; for they know that should the vulgar but be a little acquainted with their mysteries, all their juggling and knavery would be seen, and their wealth and esteem, which is the Diana they adore. That's the reason when you hear any of them cry out against me for writing physic in my mother-tongue. One holds the word of God, the other physic to be a mystery, and the vulgar must be ignorant in them both, or else will they do themselves a mischief. A learned argument![21]

Culpeper did not think much about money:

The more riches men have, the more they desire, and they never know when they have enough. For a covetous man had as many bags of gold as all those needles as Pauls would hold, and as many bags of gold as all those needles would last stitching, they would never be contended. Besides if riches consist barely in the enjoyment of money, then that man which Pliny (when Hannibal besieged Casiline, and there was a sore famine in the town) quotes, could be accounted a very rich man who sold a mouse for two hundred pence one day, and died himself for lack of food the next.

To Culpeper it did not mean much, but he was a spendthrift and despite the revenues from his many books he was always short of money.

The spirit of Culpeper lives forth in *Le Malade imaginaire* ('The Hypochodriac'), the play of Moliere. The prologue of this comedy contains a view of contemporary medicine which was shared by Culpeper:

Doctors, your learning is purely illusion,
Your remedies rubbish, your order confusion;

> Your big Latin words are unable to cure
> The sickening sadness I have to endure.
> So from my sorrow one thing is sure;
> Doctors, your learning is simply absurd.

Jean Baptiste Poquelin de Moliere (1622–1673), the famous French playwright and contempory of Culpeper, had certain traits which remind us of our hero. He suffered bitter professional jealousy of rivals, the hostility of churchman, physicians and others in the position of power. He also suffered from tuberculosis and died the night after having acted as the *malade* of his last play, the *Malade imaginaire*. In this comedy he ridicules the doctors of his time.

Beralde, the reasonable brother of the hypochondriac Argan, says:

> All you have to do is rest. Nature herself, when we let her, will take care of everything else. It's our impatience that spoils things. Most men die of their cures, and not of their diseases.
> There's two sides to your great doctors; there's what they say and what they do. To hear them talk, you'd think them the most skilful of men; to see what they do, the most ignorant. . . . Only people in perfect health have enough strength to stand up to both the disease and the cure.[22]

Moliere was *clairvoyant*, and more so than Culpeper; he not only distrusted the physicians of his time but also Mr. Purgon – the apothecary!

15

Culpeper in America

O my America, my new-found-land.

John Donne, 1571–1631

In Britain, Culpeper is undoubtedly the household name for herbal medicine, but in the United States people do not immediately associate Culpeper with herbs, although the 1983 edition of *Culpeper's Colour Herbal* is available everywhere in bookstores.[1] What people there first think of probably is the town and county of Culpeper in Virginia, the reason being that some of Nicholas Culpeper's relatives early on invested in the British Colony. Later, they became actively involved in the development and administration of the new land of the Crown.

Many gentlemen adventurers were attracted not only by the prospect of land, but by the lure of the unknown and marvellous, and by stories of fabulous riches to be won in America, which, however, only their remote descendants were to realize in ways undreamt.[2]

The first 'American' Culpepers were the brothers Thomas (1561–1613) and John (1565–1635), members of the Wigsell branch of the family. In 1609 they had invested in grants of the Virgnia Company and looked for a quick return on their money from the rapidly expanding tobacco trade.[3]

During the Civil Wars of King Charles I & II, Virginia was a colony loyal to the King and nominally under the control of the Crown. In 1648 Charles I was defeated by the general of Parliament's forces, Thomas Lord Fairfax (1612–1671). After the execution of Charles I, by English custom, his son Charles II succeeded his father. However, Parliament would not recognise him and he fled to France with his friends and supporters. Two sons of the Culpeper brothers, John first Lord Culpeper and Thomas, who originally had invested in the Virginia Company, were in exile with their monarch. For their support of the King they were given big estates in the colonies of Virginia under the charter of 1649. Unfortunately for the proprietors, while their extensive rights were clearly spelled out, it had little real value since Charles II at that time still was a monarch without a kingdom. After the restoration of the monarchy the then living Culpeper heirs, John the second Lord Culpeper, and Alexander, were finally given a new patent to their land by the General Court of Virginia in 1671.

Culpeper County and the city in Virginia owe their name to Nicholas Culpeper's relative, Lord Thomas, Colonial governor of Virginia, 1677–83. He inherited his rights from his father, John second Lord Culpeper of Leeds Castle in Kent, who held the land between the Potomac and the Rappahannock rivers in Virginia (the Northern Neck). Lord Thomas Culpeper's holdings were inherited by his daughter, Catharine, who married the fifth Lord Thomas Fairfax, descendant of the general of the Parliamentary forces in the Civil War.[4] Thus rivals on both sides of the conflict in the Civil War were united by common interests in the New World. Their son, the sixth Lord Fairfax, inherited the property. He first sent his kinsman William to manage his estates in Virginia, before he himself emigrated to America. He gave his name to Fairfax County, just outside Washington, between the Chesapeake Bay and the Blue Ridge Mountains.

Lord Fairfax was the patron of young George Washington who engaged him in 1749 at the age of 16 to survey his property. William's daughter Anne married George Washington's elder brother and his sons were close friends of Washington when he was living at Mount Vernon. It was through this alliance that the Fairfaxes were to play an important role in the development of George Washington.[4]

The town of Culpeper, Virginia, was initially called after Lord Fairfax, and later the name was changed to the present 'Culpeper'. There are also Culpepers who emigrated to the West Indies and established themselves in Barbados.[5]

Relatives of the American branch of the Culpeper family still exist today in the United States. In Virginia, the 'Medical Society of Culpeper, 1852' was founded by Drs Vernon and Charles Culpeper. In 1902 it existed in King's Daughter's Hospital, Portsmouth, Virginia.[6]

Our Nicholas Culpeper neither politically nor emotionally would have fitted into the picture of his own royalist colonial family. He was rather a part of the puritan brand of emigrants. The puritan colonists came with rebellious hearts, seeking to escape from the church-ruled government of England. These emigrants opted for the northern Commonwealth States like Massachusetts where John Winthrop in 1630 had established a thriving colony.[7]

The emigrants to the North American continent carried with them their household knowledge of skills and practices. Part of this obviously must have been Culpeper's *English Physitian*. It can be traced to the belongings of emigrants to both New England and Virginia. Moreover, two versions of Culpeper's works were actually reprinted in New England: *The English Physitian*, edited in Boston in 1708, and the *London Dispensatory*, Boston, 1720.

The Boston edition of *The English Physitian* is characteristic of the spirit of self-dependence of the New Nation. Both this and *The London Dispensatory* are remarkable documents of their time since they were the first medical books to be printed in British North America! In these publications readers found useful information for home-cure. Also the *Directory for Midwives* was an important book in the libraries of North America.[8,9]

The two Culpeper books published in Boston, Massachusetts were printed by Nicholas Boone, 'At the sign of the Bible, near the corner of School-House Lane.' The Boston edition of the *English Physitian* is a small (3 x 5 inches) publication containing only 94 pages. It obviously was intended for laymen and presented what was supposed to be Culpeper's 'choicest secrets'. The contents are arranged in alphabetical order, beginning with 'Aches, and Lameness in the Body Joynts, Limbs and Bones' and proceeding through such items as 'Bitings by Mad Dogs, Serpents', 'Childrens Infirmities' etc. The recommended remedies are for household production and largely from herbal sources. Thus for 'paines and Aches in the Back, Hip, Sides or any part of the Body', one remedy was a concoction of 'Syrup of Poppy, Syrup of Betony, and Waters of Bugloss and Sage'. The prototype of this American book was published in London in 1690 by Thomas Hawkins under the title *Physical Receips: or the New English Physician*.[9]

Culpeper's claim to fame for this masterpiece can only be associated with the spirit of its contents and the mere fact that it was attributed to a famous author known not only in England but also in America. That obviously was a selling argument and similar pirate editions are equally well known from Britain. The book did not resemble, in form or content, either the original published in 1652, or the various editions of *The English Physician Enlarged* that were subsequently printed in England.[9]

The second North American medical book also was a Culpeper. It was a reprint of Culpeper's translation of the *London Dispensatory*, published by the same enterprising Nicholas Boone in Boston, 1720. The translation was of the second edition issued by the College of Physician in 1650 and first published by Culpeper in London in 1653. It contained a premonitory epistle, 'Catalogue of Simples' (herbs), 'A Key to Galen and Hippocrates' and 'An Astrologo-Physical Discourse of the Human virtues in the Body of Man'. This book is far more important than the 1708 Boston *English Physician* since it constitutes the first American pharmacopoeia or dispensatory.[8]

It is not only a translation of the offical London Pharmacopoeia but it reflects on the personality of Culpeper in his attacks on the College and is also a revolutionary document calling for the 'Liberty of the subject' thereby well fitting into the picture of the Puritan Massachusetts.

The *English Physitian* (the *Herbal*) was the model upon which William Hughes in 1672 wrote his *American Physitian*, a compilation of herbs from the New World, mainly based on his own experience from the West Indies.[10]

A later, 1824 American edition of *Culpepper's Family Physician*, is an interesting example of the assimilation of a popular and typically English book to the New World. The editor was James Scammon of Exeter, New Hampshire, who published it with a new subtitle: 'Containing 300 medicines made of American Herbs'.[11] It is a handy pocket-sized book, very similar to the early 19th-century English editions. The main difference being that the English version specifically states '361 medicines made of English Herbs' and Scammon reduced the number to 300 because he was not sure that they actually could be found in America. Such herbs as anemone, garden arrach, birdsfoot, crosswort etc. were excluded. On the second page there is a long and detailed affidavit:

New Hampshire District, to wit:
'Be it remembered that this the 29th day of October A.D. 1824 and in the forty ninth year of Independence of the United States of America, James Scammon of the said district, hath deposited in this office the title of a book 'Culpeper's Family Physician ' . . . etc.

'. . . In conformity with the act of Congress of the United States of America . . . signed William Clagget, clerk.'

It is surprising that Scammon was awarded a copyright of Culpeper's *Herbal* with a text identical to the original, except for the omission of 61 herbs. On the other hand there was no attempt to amend this deficiency with a supplement of indigenous American herbs to make it at least appear like a genuine product of the New World. No such attempt can be traced; even the typical English scene was preserved to minute details such as: 'Roman wormwood, why Roman, seeing it grows familiarly in England'; and regarding Wild Clary: 'It grows commonly in this nation in barren places, you find it plentifully, if you look in the fields near Gray's Inn, and in the fields near Chelsea.'

Culpeper's impact on early American medicine was considerable and can be traced back to several sources. One of them is the 1696 medical note book entitled: *The Admirable Secrets of Physick and chyrurgery* by the young Massachusetts preacher and doctor, Thomas Palmer. Palmer was a family practitioner who took his job seriously and was eager to improve his knowledge. He was a self learned man who had acquired his healing art by constantly reading all kinds of books of medical authorities he could lay his hands on in New England. One of his mentors was the Mayflower doctor Samuel Fuller (1580–1633) whose notebook he had acquired. This he kept as his precious *vade mecum* and constantly kept adding his own ideas and observations to it. It is a remarkable little document since it gives to the modern reader a good picture of the state of medicine in colonial New England.[12]

Palmer frequently cites Culpeper and most of his recipes can be traced back to Culpeper's Physical Directory, but it is evident that he also was familiar with the English editions of Culpeper's *Herbal*. Both of these must have come from London since the first American editions of Culpeper's works did not appear until 1708 and 1720.

After the settlement of Australia in 1788 Culpeper's *Herbal* also was part of the baggage of the new immigrants. But it did not have the same impact as in North America because medicine had become more advanced and only a limited number of the English herbs could be found there.

16

Epilogue

New philosophy calls all in doubt;
The element of fire is quite put out;
The sun is lost, and the earth and no man's wit
Can well direct him were to look for it
And freely men confess, that this world's spent
When the planets and the firmament
They see so many new.

John Donne, 1571–1631

On Monday the tenth of January 1654 Nicholas Culpeper at the age of 38 died in his house in Spitalfields. John Gadbury relates: 'He dyed of a consumption which had been long upon him and much means was used to enervate him, but it still prevailed upon him, wasting and consuming him by degrees until it reduced him to a very skeleton, or anatomy and afterwards death released him and gave him his passport to a better world.' It was rumoured that he had been poisoned by the physicians but that could never be ascertained. Culpeper was buried in the churchyard of New Bethlehem.

Two years after Culpeper's death, on August 4, 1656, John Heydon married Alice Culpeper and moved to Spitalfields. Heydon was a mystical cheat, a professed Rosicrucian who tried many things, science, law and astrology. He had travelled widely to France, Spain and Turkey and lived above his means like a rich gentleman but was always short of money. For a time he lived in Clifford's Inn where he practised as an attorney and cast nativities. Culpeper disliked the pretentious royalist whom he had met at the Society of Astrologers in London. Several times Heydon came to visit London's best known apothecary in Spitalfields. He admired Culpeper's ability as a writer and was envious of his success because his highest ambition was to become a famous writer. In 1655 he was imprisoned by the Protector's order in Lambeth House and had his books burnt because he had foretold the date of Cromwell's death by hanging. From Heydon's writing we hear: 'I had loved a lady in Devonshire, but when I seriously perused my nativity, I found the 7th house afflicted and therefore resolved never to marry.' Although he vowed never to marry he immediately saw his chance to inherit wealth and fame when Alice Culpeper became a widow. After their marriage Heydon had no end of trouble: he fell out with many well-known authorities and was several times confined to prison because of writing treasonable matters and law-suits about money. We have reason to believe that Heydon was involved in the edition of some of Culpeper's posthumous books such as the spurious 1657: 'Mr. Culpeper's Treatise of Aurum Potabile. Being a description of the three-fold world, viz. elementary, celestial, intellectual. Containing the knowledge, necessary to the study of hermetick philosophy . . . published by his wife'

It may be of some interest to know what became of William Ryves (or Reeves), Culpeper's amanuensis who helped write his books after dictation and who eventually also wrote a short biography of his master. We meet him again in an encomium or commendation prefixed to Robert Turner's English 1656 translation of Paracelcus' strange book: *The Archidoxes of Magic*. In this he praises his friend and Paracelsus' work: 'An encomium upon his friend the translator's elaborate pains. Fly Galen hence, Hippocrates be gone; I will preserve my choice: this is the one, whose true elixir doth preserve the frame of man's frail nature, vivifies the same . . . Proceed then, friend make all speak English: why should we be barr'd our native liberty?'[1]

The book was edited by Nataniel Brook, one of Culpeper's printers who was particularly engaged in the production of esoteric texts. This indicates that Ryves after Culpeper's death became more interested in magical aspects of medicine. Otherwise there is no record of anything written by Ryves himself.

How did Culpeper fit into the cultural and scientific development of later years? 'I know very well, when I hear the cocks crow, the day is near upon breaking, this is most true that the devil is the prince of darkness, darkness the father of ignorance, ignorance the father of sin and it is the devils black boy by which he rules the world.' This is Culpeper's opinion about the cultural climate of his time.[2]

George Sarton once aptly stated: 'our views about the past are always falsified, because time has acted like a sieve, and what has been permitted to reach us is not a representative sample.'[3] Therefore only the sensational and controversial aspects of Nicholas Culpeper's life have reached us, his controversies with physicians and his views about astrology. The rest was all but buried in contemporary documents and his vast writings. I have extricated the still existing evidence about his life and character and tried to put Culpeper into perspective from the point of view of contemporary history, to highlight his influence in medicine and to clean his memory from the simplistic epithet of being a nonsensical quacksalver. The text was, however, not intended to defend the nonsense of astrological medicine.

Judgment about Nicholas Culpeper has been harsh. Charles Raven, scholar and Regius Professor of Divinity at the University of Cambridge, as late as 1947 said about him: 'a glib and largely uneducated charlatan.'[4] It is difficult to be fair to Culpeper because so little is known about him, but if we look at all that he published and read between the lines, quite a different picture emerges, and that is what I have tried to paint. It is high time that we changed our opionion about him. Today we accept Culpeper with a smile but consider him only to belong to the fringe of medicine, herbalism. Culpeper has long been unfairly judged as a superstitious quarrelsome quack because he opposed conventional school medicine at a time when it was dangerous and expensive.

It is surprising that no biography has appeared about Culpeper. The reason could not be due to a lack of significance; his life and work certainly was very exciting and has left a mark to this day. So much in fact that David Cowen said: 'The career of Nicholas Culpeper is one of the most interesting and entertaining in the history of medicines.'[5]

Some people, like the known medical historian Garrison, had no praise for Culpeper.[6] However, people who made an effort to study Culpeper, like F. N. L. Poynter, said:

> Is Culpeper worthy a study at all? May we not accept the general verdict on him as a vituperative quack who well reflects the turbulence of his times and as a founder of modern herbalist cult which flourishes at the expense of orthodox medicine? I should be content to let this verdict stand if it could be justified by the facts, but – to me at least – it seems to be so false that it might almost be characterised as 'antihistorical'. If our concern

is history of medicine as it was professed and practised, then Culpeper is a figure of outstanding importance, for he had a far greater influence on medical practice in England between 1650 and 1750 than either Harvey or Sydenham.[7]

The fact remains that biographical sources are scarce and the landmarks of his life are limited to certain dates and events. Even the entries in the *Dictionary of National Biography* are not entirely correct.[8]

Definite guidelines are offered by his publications and the colophons in his books. I have been able to trace other dates through parish registers, the Apothecaries Court Book, Sussex County Records etc. However, such details as his participation in the Civil War, his duel, and the time in Cambridge are not exactly known. The story related here about Nicholas Culpeper has therefore had to be based on ancillary information. Wherever parts were added that are not strictly supported by biographical data this has been indicated in the Notes.

Keeping in mind that an author is inseparable from his writing, it is fortunate that his books are written in a very personal style and therefore reveal facts about his life, his wife and children and their diseases as well as the conflicts with the College of Physicians etc. In addition to these facts I have tried to illuminate his fascinating life story by a juxtaposition of his contemporaries, Lilly, Harvey and Sydenham. An improved understanding is also achieved by relating his life to the historical scene of the turbulent time of the Puritan revolution and the Civil War, and by trying to give a picture of his background as revealed by the men of science and culture who influenced him: Hippocrates, Pliny, Dioscorides, Paracelsus, Bacon, Gerard and Parkinson.

If we remove the shell of mystical astrology from Culpeper's personality and work, a core of important achievements becomes evident. He clearly emerges as one of the most outstanding exponents of 17th-century medicine who was brave enough to question tradition and who contributed greatly to health education both in Britain and the New World.

Notes

Note markers in the text refer to the corresponding number in the Notes to each individual chapter but are not necessarily in sequential order in the text. Where two different note markers occur in the text, this indicates that information may be located in both citations. (*DNB* = Dictionary of National Biography, London).

CHAPTER 1:   BIRTH IN OCKLEY

1.   Harvey first presented his concept of the circulation of blood in his lectures to the Royal College of Physicians in 1616, cf. W. Harvey, *Predilectiones anatomiae Universalis* in C. D. O'Malley, F. N. L. Poynter and K. F. Russel (eds). Berkeley, 1961. The final official description came in 1628 in: *Exercitatio Anatomica de Motu Cordis et Sanguis.*

2.   According to rector Dudley Vargas, Ockley, Nicholas Culpeper, the parson of Ockley, was buried on October 5, 1616, in St Margaret's churchyard, and on October 24, 1616, Nicholas, son of the late parson was baptised in the same church. It is, therefore, very unlikely that Culpeper was 'born in London' as stated in the *DNB.*

3.   E. Parker, *Highways and Byways in Surrey*, p. 337. London, 1908.

4.   F. W. T. Attree and J. H. L. Booker, *The Sussex Colepepers, Sussex Arch Coll* 47: 47–81. 1904

5.   E. W. T. Attree and J. H. L. Booker, *The Sussex Colepepers*, Part II. *The Culpepers of Wakehurst, Sussex Arch Coll* 48: 65–98, 1905.

6.   M. F. L. Pritchard, 'The significant background of the Stuart Culpepers'. *Notes and Queries*, pp. 408–416, 1960.

7.   W. H. Blaauw, 'Wakehurst, Skaugham and Gravetye', *Sussex Arch Coll* 10: 151–167, 1858.

8.   F. N. Hepper, *Wakehurst Place. Kew Guild*, 3rd edn. Richmond, 1983.

CHAPTER 2:   YOUTH IN SUSSEX

1.   *DNB*. William Attersoll.

2.   E. Turner, Isfield Place, with notes respecting the family of Shurley. *Sussex Arch. Coll.* 18: 124–136, 1866.

3.   *Isfield Parish Register* (St Margaret) Shurley: in the parish register the name is 'Shurley', but the more common spelling later was: 'Shirley'. Other details about the Shirley, Culpeper and Attersoll families are from the same source, courtesy of the Rev. R. C. Dalling.

4.   M. Briggs, *The English Farmhouse*. London, 1953.

5.   P. Verney, *The Standard Bearer*. London, 1963, pp. 41–43.

6. D. McLean, 'Three Gentlemen Adventurers', the story of the Sherley Brothers, *Sussex County Mag.* 8: 240, 1934.
7. N. Culpeper, *The English Physitian* ('Herbal'). London, 1652.
8. M. R. Best, 'Medical use of a sixteenth-century herbal: Gervase Markham and the Banckes Herbal', *Bull. Hist. Med.* 53: 449–458, 1979.
9. J. B. Blake, 'The Compleat Housewife', *Bull. Hist. Med.* 49: 30–42, 1975.
10. N. Culpeper, *A Physical Directory* ('The London Dispensatory'). London, 1649.
11. *Architectural & Historical Guide of St. Margaret of Antioch*, Isfield.
12. N. Culpeper, *Galen's Art of Physick*. London, 1652.
13. A. R. Powys, *The English Parish Church*. London 1930.
14. Especial Observations in the last time of the pestilence. London, 1625.
15. From W. Ryves, we know that Culpeper attended a 'Free School in Sussex, but we do not know which. Lewes was a reasonable choice and so would Steyning Grammar School have been, although that was further off. About Lewes' Grammar School, cf. *History of Sussex* 2: 411–415.
16. J. Evelyn, *Diary*. Globe Edition London 1882.
17. The visit to London is not documented but was included in order to give a contemporary background.
18. G. L. Craik, *London Bridge*. In: London, C. Knight (ed.), vol. 1. pp. 73–96, London, 1851.
19. T. Vicary, *A Profitable Treatise of the Anatomie of Mans Body*. London, 1577.
20. W. Attersoll, *Three treatises: The conversion of Nineveh. Gods trumpet sounding the alarme. A sovereign remedy*. London, 1632.
21. W. Attersoll, *The New Covenant*. London, 1614.

CHAPTER 3: CAMBRIDGE AND YOUTHFUL PROTEST

1. J. Venn and J. A. Venn, *Alumni Cantabrigienses*. Cambridge 1922. According to Venn, who could not find any record of admission or degree, Culpeper started his studies in Cambridge when he was 18, i.e. in 1634. However, this is unlikely since I found a firm record of his starting as an apprentice in London in 1634. It is therefore more likely that he started at the usual age of 16, viz. in 1632. We have no record of association with any specific college, but I assume he studied at Peterhouse or Queen's where his grandfather and father, respectively, matriculated.
2. J. Milton, Cited by Raven, C. E. John Ray, *Naturalist*. Cambridge 1950.
3. J. Venn, *Early Collegiate Life*. Cambridge 1913.
4. N. Culpeper, *Culpeper's School of Physick*. London 1659.
5. J. Earle (originally published anynomously). *Microcosmography, or a peece of the world discovered*. London 1628.

6. N. Culpeper, *The English Physitian*. London 1652.
7. Everard Digby, *DNB*.
8. *Isfield*, Parish Reqister gives details about the marriage in 1624 between James Rivers and Charity Shurley, and relates the baptism of four of their children until 1629.
9. Judith Rivers, Bp 20 December, 1615. Mentioned in several of her relatives' wills. *Sussex Genealogies*.
10. James Rivers, mentioned as Esq. of Coombe in Hamsey, near Lewes. *Sussex Genealogies*.
11. C. Hole, *The English Housewife in the Seventeenth Century*. London, 1953.
12. W. Ryves, 'The Life of the admired physician and astrologer of our times, Mr. Nicholas Culpeper'. In: *Culpeper's School of Physick*. London 1659.

CHAPTER 4:   MORTAR & PESTLE

1. W. Ryves, 'The Life of the admired physician and astrologer of our times, Mr. Nicholas Culpeper'. In: *Culpeper's School of Physick*. London 1659.
2. P. Allen, 'Medical Education in 17th Century England', *J. Hist. Med.* 1: 115, 1946.
3. *Apothecaries Society, Court Book*. London 1617–1651 and information from Major Charles O'Leary. *Apothecary Society*. London, 1990.
4. S. R. Smith, 'The London apprentices as seventeenth-century adolescents'. *Past Present*, 61: 14–161, 1973.
5. We do not know if Culpeper met Pieter, but the details about Dutch whaling and scurvey-grass on Spitsbergen is documented in G. R. J. Maat, 'Human remains at the Dutch whaling stations on Spitsbergen'. In: *Early European Exploitation of the Northern Atlantic 800–1700*. University of Groningen. pp. 153–201, 1981.
6. J. Bell and T. Redwood, *Historical sketch of the progress of pharmacy in Great Britain*. London, 1880.
7. J. J. Keevil, 'The seventeenth century English medical background', *Bull. Hist. Med.* 31: 408–424, 1957.
8. R. F. Jones, *Genealogy of a classic: 'The English Physitian' of Nicholas Culpeper*. San Francisco, 1984.
9. J. G. Burnby, *A study of the English Apothecary from 1660–1760*. London, 1983.
10. J. R. Guy, 'The episcopal licensing of physicians, surgeons and midwives', *Bull. Hist. Med.* 56: 528, 1982.

CHAPTER 5:   ENCOUNTER WITH LILLY

1. N. Culpeper, *Galen's Art of Physick*. (in the introduction 'To the Reader' Culpeper mentions Lilly. The introduction was finished Oct. 20, 1651.) London, 1652.

2. W. Lilly, *Christian Astrology*. 2nd edn, London, 1659.
3. W. Lilly, *DNB*.
4. C. Hibbert, *London, The Biography of a City*, London, 1977.
5. Chambers's *Encyclopedia* Vol. 1, P.523, London, 1901.
6. W. Lilly and J. Colet, *A shorte Introduction of Grammar, for the bryngynge up of all those that entende to atteyne the knowledge of the Latin tongue, by William Lilly and John Colet*. First published in 1549 and later reprinted often until the end of the century.
7. Chambers's *Biographical Dictionary*: Donne p. 411, Edinburgh, 1936.
8. R. Burton, *The Anatomy of Melancholy*. Oxford, 1621.

CHAPTER 6: ALICE FIELD

1. N. Culpeper, *Galen's Art of Physick*, London, 1652, p. 73. Culpeper declares that he likes musik and the human voice – John Dowland (1563–1626) London musician and composer. 'Awake sweet Love' from: *The First Booke of Songes*. London, 1597.
2. W. Ryves, 'The Life of the admired Physician and Astrologer of our Times, Mr. Nicholas Culpeper'. In: *Culpeper's School of Physick*. London, 1659.
3. E. A. Parry (ed.), *Letters from Dorothy Osborne to Sir William Temple, 1652–54*. London, 1903, p. 192.
4. C. Drinker-Bowen, *Francis Bacon, the Temper of a Man*. Boston, 1963, pp. 114–115.
5. M. P. Tilley, *A Dictionary of the Proverbs in English in the Sixteenth and Seventeenth Centuries*. Ann Arbor, Michigan, 1950.
6. M. R. Holmes, *Moorfields in 1559*. London, 1963.
7. J. J. Keevil, 'The seventeenth century English medical background', *Bull. Hist. Med.* 31: 408–421, 1957.
8. J. Gerarde, *The Herbal, or Generall Historie of Plantes*. 2nd edn, T. Johnson (ed.). London, 1636.
9. N. Culpeper, *A Physical Directory*. London, 1649.
10. F. H. Garrison, *An Introduction to the History of Medicine*, 4th edn. Philadelphia, 1967.
11. N. Culpeper, *Urinalia, or a Treatise of the Crisis hapning to the Urine; Through default either of the Reins, Bladder, Yard, Conduits or Passages. With the Causes, Signs and Cures*. London, 1671.
12. N. Culpeper, *Pharmacopoeia Londinensis*, 2nd edn London, 1653.
13. J. Deacon, *Tobacco tortured*. London, 1616.
14. R. Thorius, *Hymnus Tabaci*, Leyden 1625 and London, 1651.
15. Anonymus, *A Defence of Tabacco*. London 1602.
16. E. Gardiner, *Phisicall and approved Medicines*. London, 1611.
17. N. Monardes, *Joyfull Newes out of the Newe Founde Worlde*. London, 1577.

CHAPTER 7: CIVIL WAR & FIGHTS

1. A. E. Barker, *Milton and the Puritan Dilemma*. Toronto, 1942.
2. S. R. Gardiner, *History of the Great Civil War*, vol. 1. London, 1987.
3. G. M. Trevelyan, *English Social History*. London, 1944.
4. B. Williams, *Elusive Settlement*. Walton-on-Thames, 1985.
5. J. Kenyon, *The Civil Wars of England*. London, 1988.
6. According to W. Ryves (WR. 1659), Culpeper in the beginning of the Civil War was engaged in battle and wounded, but we know of no details. In 'The English Physitian' we have records of herbs from Hatfield, St. Albans, Dunstable, Northamptom and Amersham, towns on the way from London to Edgehill where the first battle took place. The details of Culpeper's war engagement are fictitious but Harvey's presence at Edgehill is documented.
7. W. Ryves W. (WR. 1659) tells us that Culpeper was engaged in a duel and had to leave the country for some time. Details about the duel are, however, not documented.
8. R. Ollard, *Clarendon and his friends*. Oxford. 1988.
9. H. W. Haggard, *Devils, Drugs and Doctors*. Boston, 1980.
10. F. Raphael, *Byron*. London 1982.
11. N. Culpeper, *The English Physitian*. London 1652.
12. R. Crawford, *The King's Evil*. Oxford, 1911.

CHAPTER 8: PANDORA'S BOX, 1649

1. According to the *Isfield Parish Register* Elisabeth Attersoll, the daughter of A. William, minister of St. Margaret's married Anthony Parris on September 12, 1620. The visit of these relatives to London is fictitious but described in order to illustrate some aspects of Puritan life in London and Culpeper's situation when he wrote the translation of the *London Dispensatory*.
2. J. Adair, *Founding Fathers, the Puritans in England and America*. London, 1982.
3. N. Culpeper, *A Physicall Directory or a translation of the London Dispensatory* made by the Colledge of Physitians in London. London, 1649
4. W. Ryves, 'The life of the admired physician and astrologer of our times, Mr Nicholas Culpeper'. In: *Culpeper's School of Physick*. London, 1659.
5. G. Urdang, *Pharmacopoeia Londinensis of 1618*. Madison, Wisconsin, 1944 (italics of the last sentence in the text by the author); and 'The Mystery about the first English (London) Pharmacopoeia', *Bull. Hist. Med*. 12: 303–313, 1942.
6. F. N. L. Poynter, 'Nicholas Culpeper and his books', *J. Hist Med*. 17: 152–167, 1962.
7. N. Culpeper, *A Physical Directory*, 2nd edn, 1650. 1956.
8. R. F. Jones, *Genealogy of a Classic: 'The English Physitian' of Nicholas Culpeper*. San Francisco 1984.

9. W. Buchan, *Domestic Medicine*, London, 1783.
10. C. Hole, Op. cit. from: *The English Housewife in the Seventeenth Century.* London, p. 88, 1953.
11. F. G. Hofman and A. D. Hofman, *A handbook on drug and alcohol abuse.* New York. p. 45, 1975.
12. T. De Mayerne, (1573–1655) A Huguenot immigrant, court physician and Fellow of the College of Physicians, who wrote the dedication to the first Pharmacopoeia (1618) and who pioneered 'Chemical medicines' (*DNB*).
13. G. Urdang, 'How chemicals entered the official pharmacopoeias', *Arch. Int. d'Hist. Sc.* 7: 303–314,1954.
14. A. G. Debus, 'The pharmaceutical revolution of the renaissance', *Clio Med* 11: 307–317, 1976.
15. R. Le Strange, *A History of Herbal Plants.* New York, 1977. p. 134.
16. V. E. Tyler, L. R. Brady and J. E. Robbers, *Pharmacognosy.* Philadelphia, 1988, p. 492.
17. A. Huxley, *Plant and Planet.* London, 1974, p. 283.
18. J. K. Melling, *Discovering London's Guilds and Liveries.* Aylesbury, 1981.
19. J. Dobson and R. M. Walker, *Barbers and Barber-Surgeons of London.* London, 1974.
20. J. Bell and T. Redwood, *Historical sketch of the progress of pharmacy in Great Britain.* London, 1880.
21. G. Sonnedecker, *Kremer & Urdang's History of Pharmacy*, 4th edn. Philadelphia. 1976, pp. 99–104.
22. W. Brockbank, 'Sovereign remedies, a critical depreciation of the 17th century London Pharmacopoeia'. *Medical History*, 1964, pp. 1–14.

CHAPTER 9: *MIDWIFERY, 1651*

1. N. Culpeper, *A Directory for Midwives*, London, 1651.
2. N. Culpeper, *The English Physitian.* London 1652.
3. N. Culpeper, *Urinalia; or a Treatise of the Crisis hapning to the Urine; Through default either of the Reins, Bladder, Yard, Conduits or Passages. With the Causes, Signs and Cures.* London, 1671.
4. M. D. Lindheimer and A. J. Katz, 'Maternal and fetal prognosis in women with chronic renal disease'. In: *Fetal Growth Retardation*, F. A. van Assche *et al.* (eds). Edinburgh, 1981, pp. 143, 155.
5. O. Al Bahar, O. Thulesius, Johnstone and M. A. M. Hassan, 'The relationship of prostanoids to preqnancy-induced hypertension', *Int. J. Feto-Maternal Med.* 1: 2127, 1988.
6. H. W. Haggard, *Devils, Drugs and Doctors.* Boston 1980.
7. J. R. Guy, 'The episcopal licensing of physicians, surgeons and midwives', *Bull. Hist. Med.* 56: 528, 1982.
8. J. H. Baas, *The History of Medicine.* New York, 1889 (reprinted 1971 by R. E. Krieger. Huntington, New York).
9. Hugh and Peter Chamberlene, *DNB*.

10. T. Chamberlaine, *The Complete Midwife's Practice enlarged*. London 1680.
11. Friends of the University of Iowa Libraries. *Heirs of Hippocrates*. Iowa City, 1980.
12. T. Vicary, *The Englishman's Treasure, with the True Anatomy of Man's Body*. London, 1586.
13. G. Keynes, *The Life of William Harvey*. Oxford, 1978.
14. J. Dobson J and R. M. Walker, *Barbers and Barber-Surgeons of London*. London, 1979.
15. N. Culpeper, *Galen's Art of Physick*. London, 1652.
16. J. W. Harvey, *Disputations Touching the Generation of Animals*. Translated by G. Whitteridge, Oxford, 1981.
17. N. Culpeper, *Semeiotica Uranica, with a compendious treatise of urine*. London, 1655.
18. T. G. H. Drake, 'Antiques of Medical Interest: Nipple shields', *J. Hist. Med.* 1: 316, 1946.
19. J. Woodward, and D. Richards, *Health care and popular medicine in nineteenth century England*. London, 1977.
20. T. Mayerne, J. Chamberlain, and N. Culpeper, *The complete Midwifes's practice enlarged*. London, 1680.
21. J. Guillimeau, *Child-birth or, the happy delivery of women*. London, 1612.
22. A. Eccles, *Obstetrics and Gynaecology in Tudor and Stuart England*. London, 1982.
23. F. N. L. Poynter, 'Nicholas Culpeper and his books', *J. Hist Med.* 17:152–167, 1962.
24. H. Bloch, 'Nicholas Culpeper MD', *New York State J. Med.*, 1982, pp. 1865–1867.
25. J. H. Aveling, *English Midwives*. London, 1872.
26. C. Singer C. and E. A. Underwood, *A Short History of Medicine*. Oxford, 1962.

CHAPTER 10: THE HERBAL, 1652

1. N. Culpeper, *The English Physitian*. London, 1652.
2. N. Culpeper, *Galens Art of Physick*. London, 1652.
3. N. Culpeper, *Smeiotica Uranica*. London, 1651.
4. E. Sibly, *Culpeper's English Physician and Complete Herbal etc. Forming a complete Family Dispensatory and Natural System to Physic*. London, 1798.
5. *Gentlemen's Magazine*, 25: 456, 1755.
6. R. F. Jones, *Genealogy of a Classic: 'The English Physician' of Nicholas Culpeper*. University of California, San Francisco, 1984.
7. *The Weekly Intelligencer of the Commonwealth*, no. 67, 1652.
8. J. Gerard, *The Herball or Generall Historie of Plantes*. T. Jonson (ed.). London, 1633.
9. N. Culpeper, *A Physicall Directory* (translation of the 2nd edn of the *London Pharmacopoeia*). London, 1652.

10. W. Blunt, *The Art of Botanical Illustration*. London, 1950.
11. N. Culpeper, *Galen's Art of Physick*. London, 1652.
12. E. Dann, 'Kräuterbücher von der Antike bis zum Ende des Mittelalters', *Mat. Med. Nordm.* 26: 375–391, 1974.
13. B. Chance, 'Seventeenth century ophtalmology as gleaned from works of Nicholas Culpeper, physician-astrologer' (1616–1654), *J. Hist. Med.* 8: 197–209, 1953.
14. A. E. Lownes, 'The strange case of Coles vs. Culpeper', *J. NY Botanical Garden.* 41: 158–166, 1940.
15. A. Arber, *Herbals their Origin and Evolution*, 3rd edn. Cambridge, 1986, pp. 261 and 284. On p. 261 Arber refers to the 'Physical Directory' (translation of the *London Pharmacopoeia* as having the subtitle: 'Being an astro-physical discourse of the vulgar herbs of this nation'. This, however, applies to the *English Physitian* and not the *Physical Directory*.
16. N. Culpeper, *The Complete Herbal* etc. With a list of the principal diseases to which the human body is liable. London, 1824.

CHAPTER 11: WITCHCRAFT & STARCRAFT

1. *Middlesex County Records* III, 85: Culpeper, Nicholas of St. Leonard's, Shoreditch, 1642.
2. W. Notestein, *A History of Witchcraft in England from 1558 to 1718.* Washington, 1911.
3. F. King, *The cosmic influence*. New York, 1976.
4. H. G. Dick, 'Students of Physick and Astrology. A survey of astrological medicine in the age of science', *J. Hist. Med.* 1: 300–315, 1946.
5. B. Capp, *Astrology and the popular press, English almanacs 1500–1800.* London, 1979.
6. F. Bacon (translated by R. G. Gent), *Naturall and Experimental History of Winds*. London, 1653.
7. *DNB*, Digby, Sir Kenelm (1603–1665).
8. S. Partliz, *A new method of physick*. London. Translated by N. Culpeper. London, 1654.
9. T. Carlyle, *Oliver Cromwell's letters and speeches*. Part VII, p. 316. London, 1888.
10. J. Parkinson, *Paradisi in Sole, Paradisus Terrestris. Or a Garden of all Sorts of Pleasant Flowers*. London, 1629.
11. S. V. Larkey, 'Astrology and politics in the first years of Elisabeth's reign', *Bull. Inst. Hist. Med.* 3: 171–186, 1935.
12. C. Hill, *The world turned upside down*. London, 1972.
13. F. Bacon (translated by R. G. Gent), *Naturall and Experimental History of Winds*. London, 1653
14. R. Boyle, cited by P. Curry, *Prophecy and power, astrology in early modern England*. Cambridge, 1989.
15. W. Harvey, *Lectures on the whole of anatomy*. C. D. O'Malley, F. N. L. Poynter and K. F. Russel (eds). Berkeley, 1961, p. 138.

16. A. Kitson, *History and Astrology*. London, 1989.
17. N. Culpeper, *A Directory for midwives*. London, 1651.
18. N. Culpeper, *A Physical Directory*. London, 1650.
19. N. Culpeper, *Pharmacopoeia Londinensis*. London, 1654.

CHAPTER 12:   MYSTERIES OF ALCHEMY & PHYSICK

1. G. E. R. Lloyd, *Hippocratic Writings*. Harmondsworth, 1978
2. O. Temkin, *Galenism*. Ithaca, 1973.
3. N. Culpeper, *Galen's Art of Physick*. London, 1654.
4. N. Culpeper, *The English Physitian*. London, 1652.
5. J. Evelyn, *The Diary*. A. Dobson (ed.). London, 1908.
6. N. Culpeper, *A Directory for Midwives*. London, 1651.
7. N. Culpeper, In: J. Veslingius, *The Anatomy of the Body of Man*. London, 1653.
8. N. Culpeper, *A new method of physick*. London, 1656.
9. B. Chance, 'Seventeenth century opthalmology as gleaned from works of Nicholas Culpeper, Physician-astrologer (1616–1653)', *J. Hist. Med.* 4: 197, 1956.

CHAPTER 13:   PRINTED MATTERS

1. I. Walton, *The Compleat Angler, or the Contemplative Man's Recreation*. London, 1653.
2. J. Gerarde, *The Herbal, or Generall Historie of Plantes*. T. Johnson (ed.) London, 1636.
3. K. F. Russell, 'Nicholas Culpeper, his translations of Bartholin, Riolan and Vesling', *Austr. N. Z. J. Surg.* 26: 156, 1956
4. F. N. L. Poynter, 'Nicholas Culpeper and his Books', *J. Hist. Med.* 17: 152–167, 1962.
5. S. Pepys, *The Diary*. Selected and edited by R. Latham. London, 1987, p. 7.
6. M. Phelbs, *Anatomy*, catalogue 38, London, 1991.
7. W. P. D. Wightman, *Science in a Renaissance Society*. London, 1972.
8. P. Curry, *Prophecy and power, astrology in early modern England*. Cambridge, 1989.
9. N. Culpeper, *Semeiotica Uranica*. London, 1651.
10. *Council of State Papers*, November 2, 1652.
11. N. Culpeper, *Galen's Art of Physick*. London, 1651.
12. *DNB*, 'John Heydon'.
13. *Culpeper revived from the grave*. Spittafield, 1655.
14. A. Culpeper, 'Mrs Culpeper's Information, Vindication, and Testimuny concerning her Husbands Books to be published after his death'. In: *N. Culpeper, A Directory for Midwives*. London, 1656.
15. M. Mackaile, 'Culpeper's Character' in: *Moffet Well*. Edinburgh, 1664.

16. N. Culpeper, *Pharmacopoeia Londinensis*, or the *London Dispensatory*, 2nd edn. London, 1654.
17. B. Capp, 'Astrology and the popular press', *English Almanacs 1500–1800*. London, 1979.
18. *Wellcome Historical Medical Library Catalogue*. London, 1966.

CHAPTER 14: CULPEPER'S GHOST

1. G. Pliny, *Selection from letters*. C. E. Robinson (ed.). London, 1939.
2. W. H. S. Jones, *Pliny, Natural History*. London 1975.
3. W. Ryves, 'The Life of the admired physician and astrologer of our times, Mr Nicholas Culpeper'. In: *Culpeper's School of Physick*. London, 1654.
4. G. Sarton, *Six Wings*. Bloomington, 1957.
5. M. Makaile, *Moffet-Well*. Edinburgh, 1664
6. *DNB*, T. Sydenham.
7. R. Kipling, 'The story of Nicholas Culpepper'. *Lancet* ii: 5491, 1928.
8. N. Culpeper, *Pharmacopoeia Londinensis*, or *the London Dispensatory*, 2nd edn. London, 1654.
9. F. N. L. Poynter, 'Nicholas Culpeper and his books', *J. Hist. Med.* 17: 152–167, 1962.
10. F. N. L. Poynter, 'Nicholas Culpeper and the Paracelsians'. In: W. Pagel (ed.), *Science Medicine and Society in the Renaissance* 1: 201–220, New York, 1972.
11. F. H. Garrison, *History of Medicine*, 4th edn. Philadelphia, 1929, p. 289.
12. A. Arber, *Herbals*. Cambridge, 1986, p. 261.
13. W. Harvey, *Lectures on the whole of anatomy*. C. D. O'Malley, F. N. L. Poynter and K. K. Russel (eds). Berkeley, 1961, pp. 67, 89, 138.
14. B. Griggs, *Green Pharmacy*. London, 1981.
15. J. Earle, *Microcosmography* (first published anonymously in London), 1628.
16. F. H. Ellis, 'The background of the London Dispensary', *J. Hist. Med.*, July 1965.
17. N. Culpeper, *A Physical Directory*, 2nd edn. London, 1650.
18. P. Curry, 'Astrological literature in late eighteenth-century England'. In: *History and Astrology*, A. Kitson (ed.). London, 1989.
19. J. Venn, and J. A. Venn, *Alumni Cantabrigienses*. Cambridge, 1922. William Culpeper (1602–1651), son of Sir Eward Culpeper of Wakehurst was MP for East Grinstead.
20. N. Culpeper, *Catastrophe Magnatum*. London, 1652.
21. N. Culpeper, *A Directory for midwives*. London, 1651.
22. J. B. P. Moliere, *The Hypochondriac (Le Malade Imaginaire)* translated by A. Drury. London, 1988.

CHAPTER 15: CULPEPER IN AMERICA

1. *Culpeper's Colour Herbal.* D. Potterton (ed.). London and New York, 1983.
2. A. Briggs, Trevelyan, *English Social History.* London, 1978.
3. F. Harrison, *The proprietors of the Northern Neck,* Chapters of Culpeper Genealogy. *Virginia Mag. Hist. & Biography* 33: 113, 1925.
4. K. Kilmer and D. Sweig, 'The Fairfax Family'. In: *Fairfax County. Fairfax City Office of Comprehensive Planning.* Fairfax Va, 1975.
5. F. W. T. Attree and J. H. Booker, 'The Sussex Colepepers', *Sussex Arch. Collections* 47: 47–81, 1904.
6. W. B. Blanton, *Medicine in Virginia.* Richmond Va, 1933.
7. J. Adair, *Founding Fathers.* London, 1982.
8. G. Sonnedecker, *Kremer Urdang's History of Pharmacy.* Philadelphia, 1976.
9. D. L. Cowen, 'The Boston Editions of Nicholas Culpeper', *J. Hist. Med.* 2: 156–165, 1965.
10. W. Hughes, *The American Physitian.* London, 1672.
11. J. Scammon, *Culpepper's Family Physician,* containing 300 medicines, made of American Herbs. Exeter, New Hampshire, 1824.
12. T. R. Forbes, *The admirable secrets of Physick and chyrurgery by Thomas Palmer.* New Haven, Conn., 1982.

CHAPTER 16: EPILOGUE

1. Paracelsus, *Of supreme mysteries of Nature.* Translated by R. Turner, London, 1656.
2. N. Culpeper, *A Directory for midwives.* London, 1651.
3. L. Sarton, *Six Wings.* Indiana University Press. Bloomington, 1957.
4. C. Raven, *English Naturalists from Neckham to Ray.* Cambridge, 1947.
5. D. L. Cowen, 'The Boston Editions of Nicholas Culpeper'. *J. Hist. Med.* 2: 156–165, 1956.
6. F. G. Garrison, *An Introduction to the History of Medicine,* 4th edn. Philadelphia, 1968.
7. F. N. L. Poynter, 'Nicholas Culpeper and his Books', *J. Hist Med.* 17: 152–167, 1962.
8. *Dictionary of National Biography (DNB).* 'Culpeper'.

Bibliography

The best access to the works of Nicholas Culpeper is available in the London libraries of The British Museum, The Wellcome Foundation and The Royal Society of Medicine. The catalogues of these institutions (1–3) should be consulted for further studies and the bibliography of Culpeper's printed books and tracts. Another important source is the seminal work of F. N. L. Poynter, the late librarian of the Wellcome Historical Medical Library. Poynter's contribution is a paper entitled: 'Nicholas Culpeper and His Books' (4). It contains an appraisal of Culpeper's work and a list of the printed books attributed to him. The dissertation of Rex Franklin Jones puts Culpeper's *Herbal (The English Physitian)* into the perspective of contemporary herbals (5).

Here are listed the publications of Nicholas Culpeper printed during his lifetime, some which appeared after his death in 1654 and are likely to be at least partly the result of his endeavours such as translations of foreign authors with his own comments. In addition to these publications there are a number of titles which appeared under the authorship of Culpeper but whose authenticity can be disputed.

Of special interest is *Culpeper's School of Physick* of 1659 because it contains the only short biography of Nicholas Culpeper, written by his former amanuensis, W. Ryves.

I. CULPEPER'S MAIN WORKS

1. *London Pharmacopoeia.* A Physicall Directory, or a Translation of the London Dispensatory made by the College of Physitians in London . . . With many hundred additions, pp. 345 (with a portrait). London: Peter Cole, 1649. The 2nd much enlarged edition appeared in 1650. The 3rd, 1651 edition, also contains 'A Key to Galen's Method of Physick'. In all 17 editions appeared in London until 1718. Of particular interest is the American edition of the *Pharmacopoeia Londinensis* or the London Dispensatory (Boston, Mass.: Nicholas Boone, 1720). This is the second medical book to be published in North America (6).

2. *A Directory for Midwives:* or a guide for women, in their conception, bearing, and suckling their children etc., pp. 217 (with a portrait) (London: Peter Cole, 1651). The 1656 edition contains 5 plates. The book was reprinted 17 times in slightly different versions until 1777.

3. *The English Physitian:* or an astro-physical discourse of the vulgar herbs of this nation. Being a compleat method of physick, whereby a man may preserve his body in health; or cure himself, being sick, for three pence charge, with such things only as grown in England,

they being most fit for English bodies etc., pp. 259 (London: Peter Cole, 1652). This is the famous *'Culpeper's Herbal'*. Two other editions appeared in the same year, a small 12:mo with the imprint: 'Printed for the benefit of the Commonwealth of England', which Culpeper repudiated as a piracy, and a similar volume 'Printed by William Bentley'. The first American edition appeared in 1708. It has special significance since it is the first medical book published in North America (6). Its title is: *The English Physician.* Containing admirable and approved remedies for severeal of the most usual diseases. Fitted to the meanest capacity. By N. Culpeper (Boston: Nicholas Boone. 1708). More than 100 editions have been printed over the years and the latest in 1989.

II.   ANATOMICAL BOOKS

4.   *The Anatomy of the Body of Man.* Wherein is exactly described every part thereof, in the same manner as it is commonly shewed in Publick Anatomies. Published in Latin by J. Veslingius (*Syntagma Anatomicum,* Padua, 1647) and translated into English by N. Culpeper (engraved plates), pp. 192 (London: Peter Cole, 1653).

5.   *Riolan's Anatomy.* A sure guide, or the best way of physick and chyrurgery, translated by N. Culpeper and W. Ryves (London: Peter Cole, 1657). Reprinted in 1671.

6.   *Bartholinus Anatomy.* Published by N. Culpeper and A. Cole (London: Peter Cole, 1663). Reprinted 1668.

III.   OTHER MEDICAL BOOKS

7.   *A Treatise of the Rickets.* Being a disease common to children. Published in Latin by Francis Glisson, George Bate and Ahasuerus Regemorter. Enlarged, corrected and very much amended throughout the whole book by N. Culpeper, pp. 373 (London: Peter Cole, 1651).

8.   *Galens Art of Physick . . .* Translated and largely commented on by N. Culpeper (with a portrait), pp. 120 (London: Peter Cole, 1652).

9.   *A new Method of Physick.* Or a short view of Paracelsus and Galen's Practice. Written in Latin by S. Partlitius, translated into English by N. Culpeper, pp. 548 (London: Peter Cole, 1654).

10.   *Culpeper's Last Legacy.* Left and bequeathed to his dearest wife for the publick good. Containing sundry admirable experiences in severall sciences, more especially in chyrurgery and Physick (London: N. Brooke, 1655). There were 9 editions of this book, the last in 1702.

11.   *Health of the rich and poor.* In: John Praevotius, *Two books of physick.* Translated and edited by N. Culpeper. Culpeper's Ghost hereunto is added (London: Peter Cole, 1656). Reprinted until 1670.

12. *The practice of physick.* In seventeen several books. Being chiefly a translation of the works of Lazarus Rivierus. By Nicholas Culpeper, Abdiah Cole and William Rowland (London: Peter Cole, 1655). Reissued from 1661–1678.

13. *Culpeper's School of Physick.* Or the experimental practice of the whole art. The narrative of his life is prefixed (London: N. Brook, 1659). Reprinted in 1678, 1696 and 1933.

14. *Thirteen books of natural philosophy.* By Daniel Sennert and translated by Nicholas Culpeper and Abdiah Cole (London: Peter Cole, 1660).

15. *A golden practice of physick.* By Felix Plater, R. W. Abdiah Cole and Nicholas Culpeper (London: Peter Cole, 1662).

IV. ASTROLOGICAL TEXTS

16. *Semeiotica Uranica.* Or an astrological judgment of diseases etc. pp. 190 (with a portrait). (London: Nathaniell Brookes, 1651). The book was reprinted 4 times until 1792.

17. *An Ephemeris* for the year 1651, pp. 32 (London: Peter Cole).

18. *Catastrophe magnatum:* or, the fall of monarchie. A caveat to magistrates, deduced from the eclipse of the sunne, March 29, 1652. With a probable conjecture of the determination of the effects, pp. 76 (London: T. Vere & N. Brooke, 1652).

19. *An Ephemeris for the Year 1652,* being a leap-year, and a year of wonders. Prognosticating the ruine of the monarchie throughout Europe (London: T. Vere & N. Brook, 1652).

20. *An Ephemeris for the year of our Lord 1653* (London: John Macock, 1653).

REFERENCES

(1) The General Catalogue of Printed Books. The British Library. London, vol. 74. 1975.

(2) A Catalogue of Printed Books in the Wellcome Historical Medical Library. II. Books printed from 1641 to 1850. London, 1966.

(3) Catalogue of Books, Periodicals and Tracts. The Royal Society of Medicine Library.

(4) Poynter, F. N. L. Nicholas Culpeper and His Books. *J. Hist. Med.* 17:152–167. 1962.

(5) Jones, R. F., Genealogy of a Classic: *The English Physitian* of Nicholas Culpeper. Thesis. San Francisco, 1984. University Microfilms Int. Ann Arbor, 1985.

(6) Coven D. L. The Boston Editions of Nicholas Culpeper. *J. Hist Med.* 11:156–165. 1956.

Index